Testimonials

"I first met Sam not long after the family had received the diagnosis. He was a very happy and normally developing baby. I don't think we can under estimate the impact of chemotherapy and regular anaesthetics on a young child's development. When he was 3, Lisa said to me "I don't think he will ever talk."

Stress on the family and the effects of treatment slowed his development, but this was to prove to have only a short term effect on Sam.

I felt, strange as it may seem, that his development went ahead once both eyes were removed. There were no more trips to the hospital, and the uncertainty was removed. By the time he was six, I think Lisa wished he didn't talk so much!

Now there was less stress on the family, and on him, he could start to get on with his life.

It was a privilege for me to play a small part in those early years of Sam's development, and to be supporting Sam, Lisa and Jim alongside our orientation and mobility specialist, Marg Harvey and counsellor, Janet Cronin, through this very difficult time for this brave family."

Judy Reese
Early Childhood Specialist Teacher
Victorian Client Services
Vision Australia

"I first met Sam when he was enrolled in prep at the Vision Australia School. Sam was always inquisitive, wanting to know how everything worked and if it didn't, why not? His enthusiasm to learn, play and understand his environment kept many people 'on their toes' often challenging us to provide Sam with opportunities to learn while still being safe! Sam loved to climb, run, hide, play ball games and always strived to be the Winner!

Sam has an amazing sense of 'himself' when moving in both known and new environments. He is able to hear/sense cars from a great distance when waiting to cross a road. Sam uses a long cane when moving in the wider community, allowing him to move safely and independently (in those areas he has completed orientation). As Sam grows in confidence, knowledge and understanding of his community he will have the same opportunities as his siblings and peers.

Sam has a particular love of trains and I have no doubt that one day you may be travelling on the train with Sam as he is independently commuting to work, recreational activities or just to meet up with friends.

It has been a privilege to work with Sam, he has taught me many things about "having a go", motivation and the tenacity to always keep trying even if you don't succeed at first. Sam's vision impairment has not defined him nor has it deterred his drive for independence. Sam wants to have the same opportunities as his friends and to do what the other kids are doing.

Sam is fortunate to have a great, supportive and loving family. They back Sam all the way as he strives to be independent, active and happy in his life."

Gail Stinchcombe
Instructor
Orientation & Mobility
Vision Australia

"Sam's genuine love of learning and desire to learn all about the world around him make him a pleasure to teach! He has a real drive for independence and a determination to take part in every aspect of school life. Sam's tenacity and perseverance to be independent has made him 'just one of the class'."

Melissa Bowyer
Visiting Teacher
Statewide Vision Resource Centre

"I have watched Samuel grow and develop from infancy when he was diagnosed with Rb, to the impressive young man he is today – despite all the challenges that life has thrown his way so far.

He has an extraordinary knowledge of the world and maturity beyond his years. He proves to me that life is what you make of it. We have a lot to learn from the resilience of children like Samuel.

The journey Samuel has taken along with his family is indeed heart-warming and inspirational."

Sandra E. Staffieri
Retinoblastoma Care Co-ordinator
Royal Children's Hospital

"From our first contact I knew you were a family with strength! You didn't ask 'why us?' You asked, 'what can we do to help?' It was always a laugh at EUA's to see Sam running around with five Hospital Bands pinned to his back with a nappy pin! He is a fighter, a trait that can only be inherited from his parents. Lisa and Jim, you are a true inspiration for families encountering tough times, your generosity and enthusiasm to ensure families like ours take an easier path than what we experienced is a special gift. When thrown in at the deep end you can sink or swim! Thankfully we chose to swim and more importantly to teach to swim! Keep doing what you are doing, Sam is an awesome, tough, funny kid and is a credit to you! Much love the Faust Family."

Ainsley Faust
President and Founder
Beyond Sight Auxiliary RCH

"Every single person Sam comes into contact with falls in love with him and is enthralled by his wonderful zest for life. The first moment I met Sam, he took my hand and said, 'Come on, I want to give you a tour of the Starlight Express Room.' He led me past every wall and every object, explaining it all in detail

as if he could see it with his very own eyes. Now I understand how he could see it; through the eyes of his incredible imagination. I encourage you to seize this very moment and see life through Sam's eyes. His story will undoubtedly make you reflect on your own life and make you realise that life doesn't stop just because you can't see it."

Jessie Oliver
Family Relationship Coordinator
Starlight Children's Foundation

"It was January 2014 that I received a call from the Camp Quality office in regards to Companion/Camper match-ups for Middle Camp, a five-day camp for boys and girls aged between ten and twelve later in the month. The main reason for this particular call was to find out if I would be comfortable to look after a little fella who was blind. I had only been on board with Camp quality since September 2013 and, being 60, I guess it was more a courtesy call to gauge how I would feel towards the match-up. My first reaction was, well, it's not about me it's about the camper. Plus, I felt kind of proud that Camp Quality would entrust me to a boy with such special needs. That camp was where my (short, so far) journey with Sam and his family began.

Boy, was I in for the surprise of my life when first perceptions were always going to be on the cautious side, as to not want Sam to injure himself, but at the same time not want him to miss out on participating in all activities with all the other kids. Mum had packed a cane for Sam to use on camp but she may as well have packed a used bottle top because no way was that cane coming out of his bag. I stood back in total amazement throughout that camp and admired the way Sam threw himself into every challenge that was put in front of him. His willingness and ability to participate and mix with everybody on camp, Volunteers included, had to be seen to be believed. He had no disability at all – as a matter of fact in most cases he showed the way to others, proving that you can pick yourself up dust yourself off and just get on with it.

I had Sam again on the 2015 Middle Camp and nothing has changed. Sam pushes himself to the limit and is a great example of how to get the best out of himself in any situation he confronts. Sam is a normal 13-year-old boy who tests all boundaries, and sometimes crosses a few, in his enthusiasm to get things done. When needed to be reminded of those boundaries he is willing to listen and accept where he may have gone wrong. My Camp Quality journey is a short one so far but one that has been much more rewarding knowing Sam. He comes from and amazing family and I am proud to call Jim, Lisa, Sam, Mitchell and Catlin my friends. Sam, I wish you luck in everything you pursue in life, but somehow I get the feeling you are going to make your own luck, and thank you for being part of my life... I am extremely proud of you."

Sam "Ian" Grant
Volunteer
Camp Quality

"As an audio book narrator, my job is to create theatre of mind, to use the medium of sound to create a world of wonder and excitement. When you are ten years old and sound is the only form of theatre available to you, your mind becomes a boundless stage, hungry for every possible form of theatrical explosion you can throw at it. So I guess it was inevitable that Sam would find me and that one day, we would eventually meet. That day came about when his Mum Lisa contacted me and told me Sam's story. A story that immediately resonated. A story of courage, determination and a compelling desire to live life full of joy and happiness – traits rare in anyone so young, but particularly unique in a kid who had already faced such monstrous hurdles. You can't help but be inspired by Sam. He and I are kindred spirits, unlikely buddies that share a love of the absurd and a desire to make people laugh. I hope Sam will always be a part of my life. I look forward to following his journey into adulthood and one day, I will be watching him accept some award, or make some speech or solve some global problem, I will sit back proudly and say, 'Yep, I knew him when he was a kid.'"

Stig Wemyss
Audio Book Narrator, Writer, Director, Producer
Mezzanine Productions

"Jim and Lisa's story will emotionally move you, inspire you and ignite your passion for living life to the fullest!

It's a story that makes you grateful for all that you have and teaches us about courage and what it takes to be successful."

Darren J Stephens
#1 International Bestselling & Author of
Millionaire & Billionaires – Secrets Revealed

Life THROUGH Sam's Eyes

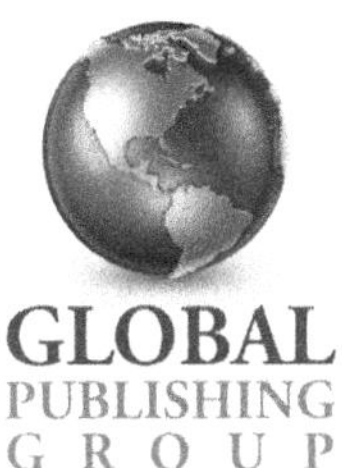

Global Publishing Group
Australia • New Zealand • Singapore • America • London

Life THROUGH Sam's Eyes

How Our Blind Son Helped Us See...

Jim and Lisa Valavanis

DISCLAIMER

All the information, techniques, skills and concepts contained within this publication are of the nature of general comment only and are not in any way recommended as individual advice. The intent is to offer a variety of information to provide a wider range of choices now and in the future, recognising that we all have widely diverse circumstances and viewpoints. Should any reader choose to make use of the information contained herein, this is their decision, and the contributors (and their companies), authors and publishers do not assume any responsibilities whatsoever under any condition or circumstances. It is recommended that the reader obtain their own independent advice.

First Edition 2016

National Library of Australia
Cataloguing-in-Publication entry:

Creator: Valavanis, Jim, author.

Life Through Sam's Eyes : How Our Blind Son Helped Us See / Jim Valavanis ; Lisa Valavanis.

1st ed.
ISBN: 9781922118677 (paperback)

Blind children – Home care – Australia.
Children with disabilities – Australia – Family relationships.
Parent and child –Australia.
Positive psychology.

Other Creators/Contributors:
Valavanis, Lisa, author.

Dewey Number: 649.151

Published by Global Publishing Group
PO Box 517 Mt Evelyn, Victoria 3796 Australia
Email info@GlobalPublishingGroup.com.au

For further information about orders:
Phone: +61 3 9739 4686 or Fax +61 3 8648 6871

We dedicate this book to our inspirational son Sam, who has come into our lives to teach us about courage, strength, resilience and unconditional love.

This book is also dedicated to our family and friends, who have supported us through the very difficult emotional times and given us the strength to fight for Sam's health and wellbeing.

Jim and Lisa Valavanis

Acknowledgements

It has been an amazing experience to be able to write this book with Jim and tell our family's story. We would not have been able to survive the last thirteen years of our lives without a lot of help, love and support from many wonderful people. It is because of them that this book has evolved. We would like to take this opportunity to say "Thank You".

Firstly, thanks go to our amazing family, whose strength has helped us fight many battles.

To my parents, Joy and Darrel Polglase. You spent many, many hours in the waiting and recovery areas of the Royal Children's Hospital, Peter MacCallum Cancer Institute and Royal Victorian Eye and Ear Hospital with me. You saw and experienced things that a grandparent shouldn't have to. You were there for Sam, but more for me. I love you both very much.

To Mum. You weren't here to see this book come to fruition. I miss you very much, but know that you will always be there for me and us.

To Jim's parents, Stella and Angelo Valavanis. Through the hard times and beyond you have always been there with love and support.

To Jim's brother and his wife, Paul and Sofie Valavanis, and their children Nicholas, Christian, Alex, and Cleo. Thanks for an ear and shoulder when we needed it.

To all of our amazing friends who have seen us through part or all of this journey. You have been there with meals at the end of an exhausting chemotherapy day, a night out when the insanity gets too much and boxes of tissues and chocolates when we needed them.

To all of the medical staff at the Royal Children's Hospital Melbourne, Peter MacCallum Cancer Institute and Royal Victorian Eye and Ear Hospital who have helped us along the way. You showed compassion and respect towards us as parents. We never felt like Sam was just another patient.

Ophthalmologists Dr John McKenzie and Dr James Elder, Chemotherapy Oncologist Dr John Heath and Radiation Oncologist Dr Greg Wheeler. What do you say to people who are responsible for saving your son's life? Thank you.

Orthoptist Sandra Staffieri. What you do is not just a job for you. As with all the other 'Rb' families, you were there for us with guidance, support and friendship. You were always there to join us for the happy or sad tears. I know you take on all of our traumas as though they were your own. But I cannot imagine anybody else to have been able to help us through the last thirteen years. Thank you.

Thanks to the very talented Ocularist, Patrick Loyer. You are an amazing artist who has the ability to trick people into thinking that Sam can see. The prosthetic eyes that you created look more realistic and beautiful than Sam's treatment damaged real eyes ever did. And the best part is, his prosthetic eyes cannot get cancer in them!

To all of the other 'Rb' families and their strong, courageous children. You are the group of people who say "I understand", and you really do. We are all there to support each other through the highs and lows.

The Beyond Sight Auxiliary, formed by a couple of selfless 'Rb' families. Without the support and fundraising of Beyond Sight, Sam's diagnosis and treatment may have been very different. We are proud to have been able to help raise funds and awareness for this little known childhood cancer through Beyond Sight.

A big thanks goes to the unbelievable charities and volunteers who do an amazing job of getting sick kids through the hard times and beyond, giving them a sense of fun, adventure and acceptance. But importantly they are also there for the siblings and families of these kids. Thanks to them, we have been personally involved in fun days, kids and family camps, Christmas parties, weeks/weekends away as a family and adventures beyond our wildest dreams. Thanks to Starlight Children's Foundation, Camp Quality, Challenge, Ronald McDonald House Charities and Rotary Club Noble Park. To all the volunteers who give from the heart, thank you.

To *The Today Show*, Channel 9, and wonderful friends Rebecca and Brendan Bishop. Thanks for a once in a lifetime trip to Disneyland a month before Sam lost his sight. This will be a visual memory for him always. Most definitely it is the "Happiest Place on Earth".

To the Rotary Club, Noble Park. Thanks to Ron Damon and all of the wonderful members who brightened our lives with a holiday to the Gold Coast, Queensland, to visit the Theme Parks and have family fun in the sun.

Thanks to Vision Australia (formerly RVIB). You have helped, guided, educated and supported us from the start and will be there for the rest of Sam's life.

Special thanks goes to Judy Reese, Marg Harvey, Gail Stinchcombe, Garry Stinchcombe, The Vision Australia School, Feelix Library, the Orientation and Mobility Department, the Early Childhood Education Department, Occupational Therapy Department, Physiotherapy Department, Music Therapy Department, Blind Sports Victoria and all the other people and Departments who have helped us over the years, too numerous to list, but you know who you are.

To Statewide Vision Resource Centre, who help Sam to learn many skills that sighted people take for granted.

To his amazing visiting teacher, Melissa Bowyer, who visits Sam twice a week at school. You have been an incredible source of help and support to both Sam and us. I cannot thank you enough for all that you have done for Sam.

To Maria Elford, thanks for fuelling Sam's love of geography with the tactile maps.

To the staff and supporters of Guide Dogs Victoria for their amazing Orientation and Mobility camps. The more fun Sam has, the more he seems to learn and grow in confidence.

Thanks go to Patterson Lakes Kindergarten. Four-year-old's kinder can be a tricky enough year, with the transition to school looming ahead. Sam lost his sight part way into this important year. It is due to the wonderful staff that this was handled as calmly and with the greatest amount of care that it could have been. Thanks to Sue, Karen and Jenny, who were wonderful to Sam and also to Jim and me. You helped a life changing event be as emotionally pain free for Sam with his peers as possible, making the result a new "normal" for this kinder kid.

A huge thank you must go to Berwick Chase Primary School, with special mention to Principal Murray Geddes. Murray, from before the school even existed, you have been determined that whatever Sam needed to be included as a regular student, you would make sure it was provided for him. You have been supportive of Sam and the rest of our family to make Sam's transition from the Vision Australia School to Berwick Chase Primary School as smooth as possible. You have never looked at Sam as a disabled student, but have taken the same nurturing and supportive approach to Sam as you do with all of your students, instilling in him a sense of confidence, determination and a love of learning. All of these traits that will see him achieve great things as a blind adult, in what can be a discriminating sighted world.

Thanks also to all of the staff who have had the pleasure of teaching our son, and fuelling his thirst for knowledge and information. To the teachers and integration aids, you have helped to shape Sam into the young man he is today. Thank you all.

To Daphne Proietto, whose talent is inspiring. Your patience in teaching Sam piano was incredible. Thanks for what you have done for Sam on and off the piano.

A big thanks goes to Sam's heroes, although unaware of who Sam is, you have changed his life. Andy Griffiths, Terry Denton, Paul Jennings and Morris Gleitzman. And also to Stig Wemyss, who Sam idolises and has had the privilege of meeting. Through Bolinda Audio, your wonderful adventures have come to life and sparked a love of storytelling and reading in Sam.

To all the people who have inspired Jim and I through their courage, strength and determination. Janet Shaw, Stevie Wonder, Andrea Bocelli, Ray Charles, Ben Underwood, Erik Weihenmayer, Gerrard Gosens, Ched Towns, Helen Keller, Jeff Healey, Nick Vujicic, Kurt Fearnley, Paul de Gelder, Turia Pitt, Jim Stynes, Christopher Reeve.

And to those who make us want to grab all that life has to offer and be better people for it. Pat Mesiti, Dr John Demartini, Dr Wayne Dyer, John Gray, Sir Richard Branson, Anthony Robbins, Robert Kiyosaki, Stephen R. Covey, Brian Tracy, Zig Ziglar, Mark Victor Hansen, Jack Canfield, Jim Rohn, Dale Carnegie, Napoleon Hill, John Ilhan, Peter Walsh.

A huge thanks goes to Darren J Stephens and Jackie Tallentyre. You took us under your wing and helped us beyond words. You made us Authors. But more importantly, you showed us our worth and value as parents. Without you there would be no book.

To my wonderful husband Jim. You have always been there for me and our three beautiful children Samuel, Mitchell and Caitlin. Although times have been very hard and we have faced our darkness differently, I know that you are there beside me all the time. Forever and three days.

To my 'twins born five years apart', Mitchell and Caitlin. You have both brightened my life in what have been some not so happy times. You both wouldn't admit it, but you love your big brother very much and would do anything to help and protect him. You have shown me what a real childhood without sickness is meant to be. I love you very much, my two little monkeys.

And finally, to my son Sam. You have changed my life in so many ways. As with all families, we have our good and bad times. We have both threatened to run away, but who else would have us? You are my son, my friend, my teacher, my mentor, my inspiration and my life. I love you very much, Sam. Love from Mummy (and Daddy).

FREE BONUS GIFTS

Exclusive Interviews, Checklists & Relaxation Music

Valued at $297

Claim your FREE BONUS GIFTS by going to…

www.LifeThroughSamsEyes.com/Bonuses

Instant Access and FREE Download

As a way of saying thank you for investing in our book, we would like to reward you with some very special gifts.

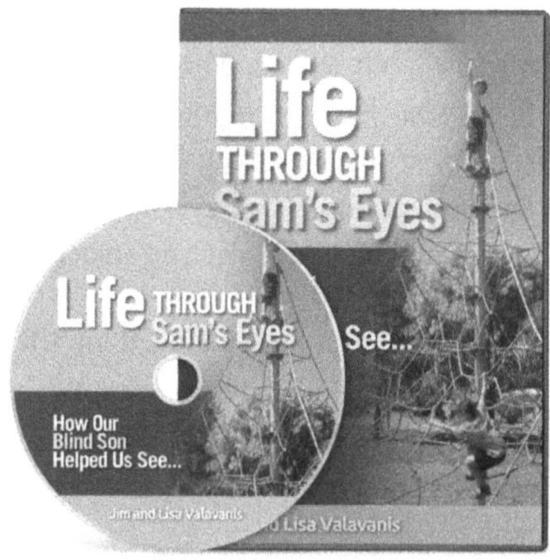

Claim your FREE BONUS GIFTS Valued at $297 NOW by going to… www.LifeThroughSamsEyes.com/Bonuses

Contents

Foreword

All we ever truly want for our children is for them to be happy and healthy – anything else is a bonus. However, every minute of every day a child is admitted to hospital somewhere in Australia and for thousands of these families what comes next is a diagnosis that changes the life of the child and the family forever.

Sam and his family are one such family and they have provided much inspiration for all of us at Starlight.

At Starlight we have a range of programs to support the wellbeing and resilience of seriously ill children and their families by transforming their experience of hospitalisation and treatment.

Originally, Starlight granted children their life changing Starlight Wish, but over the years we recognised the real need for these children and their families to also have support in the hospital environment. The wards were clinical and often scary for the children. Now in every major paediatric hospital in Australia Starlight provides a haven away from the stress and pain of treatment through our Starlight Express Rooms and our amazing Superhero, Captain Starlight. For me to watch a child, clearly in pain and stressed, wheeled into a Starlight Express Room and to see that child's head lift as they take in this new and fun place and then, 20 minutes later, roaring with laughter and forgetting their IV drip or other medication...that is the transformation Starlight delivers seven days each week.

Starlight's Fun Centre program is available in over 100 hospitals nationally and Starlight is the only organisation with a permanent presence in every major paediatric hospital around the country with programs available every day. In addition, a Starlight Wish is granted every day.

While Sam was in hospital he loved the distraction provided by the Starlight Fun Centres and he loved to spend time in the Starlight Express Room. Sam was one of the many 'favourites' of our Captain Starlights.

In fact, Sam and his family chose to spend their final moments together before his operation having fun in the Starlight Express Room.

But Sam's operation was no ordinary operation. Imagine being told your child was to lose an eye to cancer. For Sam's family this had been devastating enough. Imagine then being told that Sam's remaining eye also had a tumour and had to be removed. This is the news Sam's family had to accept – this was their new reality.

When I heard that the Starlight Express Room was the place Sam and his family chose to spend those final moments before the operation – that the Starlight Express Room and Captain Starlight was one of the last things Sam would ever see, I was overwhelmed. To me it was a wonderful demonstration of the impact of our Starlight programs and of Starlight's ability to provide families with positive memories that last forever.

Sam and his family have been supported by some great examples of Starlight fun and distractive therapy and over the years they have been involved in our Starlight activities like visits to the zoo, weekend breaks, chocolate festivals and a family trip to the Royal Melbourne Show. Activities that other families often take for granted but are a special treat for families with seriously ill children.

Sam and his family, including his little brother Mitchell and little sister Caitlin, enjoy life for all it has to offer and Sam is always sporting the biggest smile in the world.

The support Starlight provides is considered by the hospitals to be integral to the total care of the child. However, it is not just the seriously ill child who benefits but the entire family – especially siblings like Mitchell and Caitlin who often spend enormous amounts of time in hospital. Siblings and the entire family are warmly welcomed to be involved in our Starlight activities in and out of hospital.

The need for us to support these children and their families everyday means we need funds to deliver our Starlight programs every day.

At Starlight we are incredibly proud to be part of Sam's journey. We thank Sam and his family for making Starlight the beneficiary of the proceeds from the sale of this book and we hope it is an amazing success.

Louise Baxter
Chief Executive
Starlight Children's Foundation

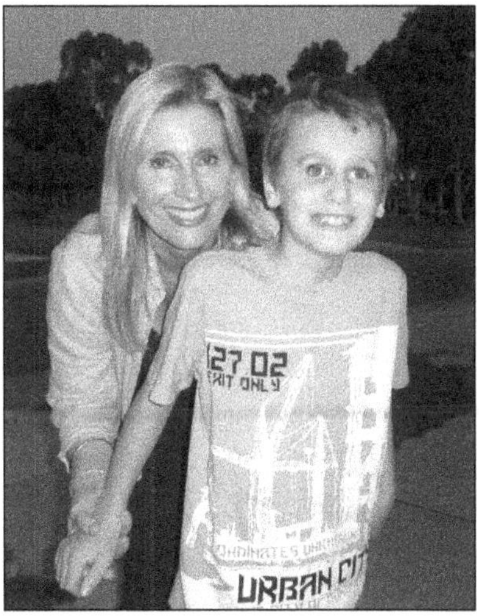

Introduction - A Dad's Perspective

(Jim)

When it was dark now there's light
Where there was pain now there's joy
Where there was weakness I found strength
All in the eyes of a boy

Celine Dion – 'A New Day Has Come'

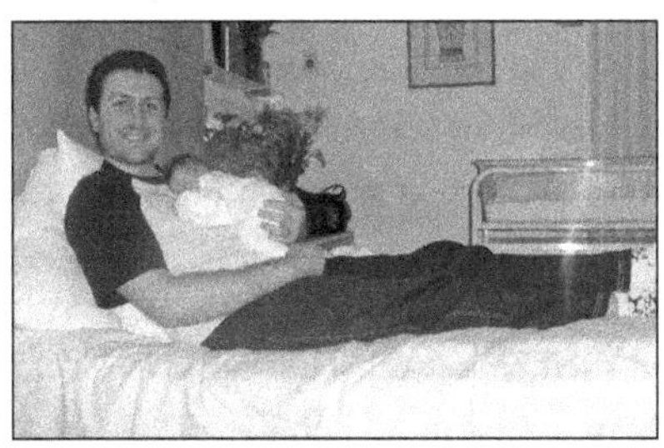

It was the proudest moment of my life on Christmas Eve in 2001, when Lisa told me that we were going to be parents for the first time. We had always discussed having a family and how it would change our lives and bring us even closer together. Little did we know at the time, but in less than twelve months our whole world would be turned upside down.

Sam entered the world at 2:37 pm on the 30th August 2002. It was a very difficult delivery, to say the least. A two-day long labour had taken its toll on Lisa, who was extremely exhausted and numb from the waist down. Sam didn't want to pass through the birth canal very easily and his heart rate had dropped, so medical intervention was required. This was by way of vacuum extraction and forceps, which was quite traumatic for a first time father to witness. I was a pall bearer at a friend's funeral the day of the birth so it had been an emotional rollercoaster.

I cut the umbilical cord. The gruelling, long hours endured were all worthwhile. It was great to hear Sam let out his first cry, and I sighed with relief knowing he was out safely. I can still remember the warm fuzzy feeling which came over me when I thought about the miracle of life that we had just created, and all the happy memories we would make together in the future.

I wanted to enjoy every little special moment and promised myself that I would be a very 'hands-on' dad, from feeding to bathing to changing nappies. Life couldn't get any better, but that was all about to change.

At six weeks we had noticed that Sam wasn't hitting the milestones like the other babies in the mother's group. Sam would not look at us directly in the eyes and they would flicker around uncontrollably to the light and not focus on one particular thing. We were concerned as first time parents and wanted answers.

We first saw a Chiropractor, that told us Sam may possibly have a brain stem injury and would need further testing. This came as a total shock to us and we didn't know who to turn to or what to do next.

We went for our post-natal follow up examination with our Paediatrician, who tried to reassure us that a newborn's sight could take up to twelve weeks to fully develop and we shouldn't be too worried. We had a gut feeling that something wasn't quite right, but we trusted the doctor and went away feeling we needed more information.

Whilst nursing Sam one night, his pupils were fully dilated and I noticed a milky white mass in the back of his eyes when the light from the lamp shone in at certain angles. It didn't look "normal" or sit well with me.

Our next visit with the Maternal Child Healthcare Nurse confirmed that there was some cause for concern, as he wasn't following the visual cues that a baby of his age should. She had been concerned about Sam for a while, but wasn't able to pinpoint exactly what was wrong. She also said that a mother knows best when it comes to their child, so she rang our Paediatrician for a referral to a Paediatric Ophthalmologist. As he still didn't seem overly concerned and pretty much brushed us off, he gave her the details to contact the specialist herself. We were then booked in for the next available date.

I can still remember the nervous tension we were feeling in anticipation of the news. We were called in to the room and after further testing and assessment told in no uncertain terms, that our son's retinas were detached and that he was more than likely going to be blind and could possibly have cancer. I was numb and speechless, feeling like our world as we knew it had come crashing down around us, and that someone had reached their hand into my chest and ripped my heart out.

We left there feeling helpless and contemplating our future with a newborn who was blind and could possibly have cancer. This came completely from left field. Who could we turn to? What were we going to do?

Two days later we were in at the Royal Children's Hospital in Melbourne having all the necessary tests, including a lumbar puncture to diagnose his condition. Our worst nightmare was confirmed. His retinas were detached and he did have 'the C word', which was a very rare childhood cancer called retinoblastoma. Lisa recalls the first words from my mouth when we found out. "That's just killed me!" We'd never heard of it before nor knew anyone that had this condition. How could it be that a baby is born with cancer?

As first time parents it should have been an incredible and joyous experience, but that couldn't have been further from the truth. We felt so alone and isolated whilst we sat in the waiting room at the Royal Children's Hospital and wept doing our best to console each other, as we tried to envisage our child's future and what lay ahead for us. It was the scariest day of our lives, but we were in the best place to tackle it head on.

He had surgery in the coming days to insert a Hickman line for the chemotherapy treatment, which began almost immediately. We didn't even have time to think about it. It was hard to imagine poison coursing through his tiny veins. He took it all in his stride, enduring month after month of long hospital visits and stays.

Once a month, we would get to hospital around midday and had to sit in the waiting area till 5 or 6 pm to get an update on the tumours through an examination under anaesthetic, using a RetCam (this was a special camera that the Ophthalmologists used to take photos of the eyes and track the disease's progress). We had knots in our stomach till we were given the news by the doctors at the end of the day. We couldn't feed him from 7 am onwards due to the fact that we had to fast him for the anaesthetic. You can't reason with a hungry three- to six-month-old baby.

Sam had countless GAs (general anaesthetics) for examination under anaesthetic (EUA). We believe it was well over 100 GAs in total. He found it very difficult to go under anaesthetic intravenously (by a needle) and he would kick and scream frantically. Can you blame him? We found that the best way to put him to sleep was to use a face mask and place some chocolate smelling essence around the edge of it. He later named this the 'chocolate mask' and would always ask for it. This caused far less stress for all involved in the process, even though some Anaesthetists from time to time would insist he was too old for the mask. They soon found out why we chose to go down this path!

His treatments were gruelling, and this went on for four and a half years. First off there was chemotherapy, which was given to him intravenously in the Day Chemo Ward of the old Royal Children's Hospital. It wasn't a very pleasant environment for the children or the families, and every now and then you would hear someone vomiting or crying uncontrollably. He had quite a number of rounds and it worked to some extent, but it wasn't enough to stop the cancer entirely. There was only so much chemotherapy that he could be given before the levels became dangerous to his health.

He also had cryotherapy (liquid nitrogen), which looked like he'd gone ten rounds with Mike Tyson. It was described to us like frostbite and must have been extremely painful and uncomfortable for Sam. This treatment was followed up with eye drops to help with managing the pain and to stop infection. This would take the two of us to get them into his inflamed eyes and was emotionally very difficult to do. We had to pin him down to administer the drops and antibiotics while he was thrashing about.

The least invasive treatment he had was laser therapy. It was described to us like having sunburn and was useful in getting rid of the smaller cancer cells which were towards the front of the eye. He bounced back a lot quicker after having this treatment and it would give us comfort in knowing that the cancer was under control for another month, at least until the next follow up.

Then there was the radiation at the Peter MacCallum Cancer Institute. This was an intense treatment which went for four weeks and we would have to go in each morning from Monday to Friday during this period.

When I wasn't able to go in, Lisa's parents would join her for moral support. This treatment was again done under a general anaesthetic and he had to have a special fibreglass mask made to keep his head perfectly still, because the radiation given was done so with pinpoint accuracy to the targeted area. This treatment was the most difficult for me to sign off on, because we were told that there may be long term side effects from this such as bone malformation and possibly secondary bone cancer in the future.

We were then off to the Royal Victorian Eye and Ear Hospital where he had radioactive plaques inserted into his eyes on three separate occasions. An incision was made in his eye and the plaque was left in there to do its thing for a few days, then removed. We were advised by the staff at the hospital not to go within a metre of him whilst the plaque was in place, but how can you not cuddle or be close to a child that is in pain and discomfort.

The last treatment that was suggested to us by the doctors when all else had failed was chemotherapy injections directly into the eye. This had never been tried before at the Royal Children's Hospital, but they were out of alternatives and even spoke to specialists overseas for some new protocols and advice on how to handle it. Sam had a few of these treatments following lengthy discussions and with us weighing up all the options.

We had explored every possible treatment option there was, even trying methods that hadn't been performed before in Australia. But we were in very good hands and trusted them implicitly knowing that they would do the very best for our son. The Royal Children's Hospital Melbourne is one of the world leaders in retinoblastoma diagnosis and treatment and the use of the RetCam has certainly come a long way from how they previously tracked the disease by drawing the tumours on a piece of paper.

After we removed his left eye at the age of three, the right eye which had been dormant for 15 months started getting active tumours popping up in it again. His vision was very poor to begin with, having had no central vision, only peripheral, but it was enough to help him get around and be independently mobile. It was described to us by the doctors as if you are holding a fist up in front of your eye and you can only see the surrounds.

It felt as though the nightmare had started all over again, just when we thought we were on top of it. We couldn't cut a break. The treatment went on for many months and we couldn't see the light at the end of the tunnel.

We can honestly say that we tried absolutely everything to save Sam's sight, but in the end it was not meant to be. The most important thing of all is that we still have Sam in our lives and we hope that what we subjected him to in the formative years of his life will not have a negative impact on his long term health and wellbeing.

Lisa got in touch with Vision Australia the day after we were delivered the savage blow that our son could possibly be blind or have a significant vision impairment. I got onto the internet and started researching retinoblastoma. This wasn't a great idea in my fragile state, as I read some horrific stories and outcomes.

We were put in touch with Ainsley, Stuart, Sarah and Mark who had started up the Beyond Sight Auxiliary and Parent Support Group at the Royal Children's Hospital. This group provides support to parents that have children diagnosed with retinoblastoma and was a great support network for us to meet at the time.

We were invited to the Kew Traffic School by Beyond Sight, where we met other families who had travelled down the same road, which helped us realise that we were not alone in our battle. We could discuss all of our fears and uncertainties and put our minds at ease for the time being.

We were living month to month between hospital visits… it became like our second home. It was all a blur at the time and we couldn't see a future. We were so consumed with Sam's treatment and getting him better that nothing else mattered. It made us reassess our lives and put everything else into perspective. People complaining about trivial things made no sense to us at all. We had much bigger things to worry about.

This had a major impact on my life with significant consequences. I withdrew from society and I didn't want to leave the house, see anyone nor speak to anyone. When I did go out, I would put on a brave face and a fake smile so it appeared that I was in control. After all, men don't show their emotions!

I spiralled further and further into a deep depression but still wouldn't admit it to myself. Lisa would encourage me to seek professional help, but I was a 'man' and I could deal with it on my own, or so I thought.

I got on with life because I had to. I felt like I had no other choice. I was the man of the house and the breadwinner and Lisa had to take care of Sam's needs at the time. I had to provide for my family and give them a safe and secure environment. We, as men, are in society's eyes the provider and the protector.

I needed time out. I just wanted to jump in my car and drive as far away as I could. I felt like I couldn't share this with anyone because it would show a sign of weakness. Luckily I was able to take my long service leave with the employer I had been with for ten years. I engrossed myself into landscaping our backyard with the help of my father. This provided solace for me and I was able to focus my attention on something other than the real issues we were dealing with on a day to day basis.

After a few months off and plenty of time to think, it wasn't getting any better. I tried to fix things by changing my environment, but in the end it didn't really help. I studied a few courses, changed jobs a number of times and even gave my own business a go. This didn't end very well and unfortunately also ended a 25-year friendship, as I went into partnership with my best friend.

We were offered counselling and the opportunity to get involved with various charity groups which involved family days and escapes, so that we could mix with other families that were going through similar experiences to us and share our stories, but also as a chance to forget about our cares for a little moment in time.

In the beginning I found it very difficult to accept these offers, as I felt that I couldn't have fun or enjoyment in my life when my son was going through hell on earth and having gruelling surgeries and treatments every month. I felt enormous guilt.

I tried to speak to counsellors and psychologists on a number of occasions, but that would bring up all the bad memories over and over again that I was trying to suppress. If I could offer one word of advice here, this is exactly what you should be doing. Don't hold it in, as it not only prolongs your recovery, but keeps you in a very dark place. Get it out!

I also found it difficult going to playgrounds, parks and public places that had big groups of children, because everywhere I looked there were 'normal' kids. It would make me think ahead to the times where I wouldn't be able to kick a footy, play cricket or golf, ride a bike etc. as these were activities I enjoyed. I now know, that I was only thinking of the things I couldn't do, rather than the things I could do. These were pretty dark times and I could only focus on the negatives rather than the positives.

We put off having a second child until we got our genetics' tests back. It took about nine or ten months and had to be sent to Adelaide because that's where they were conducted. They came back all clear! We couldn't put another child through what Sam had endured. However, in saying that, if he chooses to have any children, there is a 50% chance that his kids will have the condition, because he is a carrier. That is all ahead of us and we will cross that bridge when we come to it. Apparently it was a freak of Mother Nature, a genetic mutation which can happen to anyone. We were unlucky enough to draw the short straw.

I felt like I couldn't start living again until I knew that my son was in the clear. I now know that it wasn't healthy for me or my family to be in this state of mind, but that's just how I felt at the time. It was holding me back and I refused to make any plans for the future.

Whether you are a spiritual person or not, I truly believe that things happen for a reason and you are never given more than what you can deal with. This has taken me a long time to come to terms with, but I can confidently say that I am now at peace. This has changed us as individuals and as a couple, making us stronger and bringing us closer together. We know many couples that have gone their separate ways due to the enormous stresses and pressures that come with having a sick child.

Having Mitchell when we did was a very special gift. He came at the right time in our lives which helped us move on and get back a sense of normality, which we craved more than anything. In saying that, for some unusual reason I showed resentment towards Mitchell because there was nothing wrong with him. I don't know where these feelings and emotions came from. All we had known up until that point as parents was hospital visits, ongoing treatment and check-ups. I remember thinking to myself, "There must be something wrong with him". I would look for flaws and faults which weren't there. He was PERFECT!

He is a beautiful, charismatic boy, with loads of personality who makes us laugh every day. He was sent to us to help us look at the bright side of life and to begin living again. He has brought joy and happiness into our lives and we welcome the future with open arms. I can also say the same about the youngest member of our family, our gorgeous princess Caitlin who is wise beyond her years, but so sweet and innocent just the same.

When Sam lost his sight, I wanted to understand what he was going through and what he was dealing with, so I would close my eyes and walk around the house like a blind man with my arms out in front of me feeling for objects so I wouldn't bump into them. This really hit home as to what lay ahead for Sam and I struggled with the idea of him living his life in darkness.

Before Sam lost his sight I would play 'feely' games with him, to make him become aware of his surrounds and help him adjust to life without sight. I would get him to close his eyes and feel the foam letters of the alphabet along with numbers whilst in the bath tub and memorise how they felt and their overall shape. We would then spell words out of the letters to make a game of it. Sam also loved Thomas the Tank Engine and in no time at all had memorised each and every character that he possessed by touch. It surprised me how quickly he had picked it up. In a way, it put my mind at ease knowing he would be okay in the future. This gave me the hope and encouragement that he would be more than capable of handling life with a vision impairment.

Sam will quite often say, "I wish I could see mum/dad". He has his good and bad days, which is understandable.

We all have choices in life, but sometimes those choices are made for you. I felt extreme guilt for a long time that we had blinded our child and totally changed the course of his life. We should be the ones that protect and nurture him from all the bad in the world. It took me a very long time to get out of this headspace and accept that the decision we had made was for our son's long term health and welfare. It had felt like the 'death of his sight'.

It was time to move on from grieving and mourning the loss of his sight and think of it as a new beginning, with new challenges. I had to shift my way of thinking from what we didn't have, to what we did have. We had the most important thing in our lives… our son. I could still hug and kiss him, talk and laugh with him and share many wonderful experiences with him. That was all ahead of us. We could make new memories to "look" back on.

I can still recall the nauseous feeling in the pit of my stomach and the lump in my throat on the morning of the day we were due to go in to hospital for Sam's surgery to remove his remaining eye. It was really going to test us as a couple and as a family and we all needed to be there to support each other through this very traumatic event.

It was like a dream, like I was having an out of body experience looking down on the whole family, who was still trying to come to terms with the fact that once Sam had come back into recovery from theatre he would be blind. Luckily we had the Starlight Express Room downstairs to distract us for a little while and to meet Captain Starlight and the other staff in there, who bring smiles, joy and laughter to children all over the country.

Lisa and I both tried to keep a brave face for the rest of the family, but just beneath the surface was a couple of very scared and uncertain individuals of what lay ahead for our brave little boy who was still under general anaesthetic.

When he was brought out of theatre he was still unconscious from the general anaesthetic, and Lisa and I were both there to be with him when he woke up. He would normally come out of an anaesthetic quite angry and aggressive, but this time it was different. He was very groggy and kept asking when he could see again. This was devastating to hear as a parent and we had explained to him beforehand that he would not be able to see with his eyes again, but would instead be able to 'see' with his hands and ears.

We stayed in hospital overnight for monitoring and to ensure that there were no complications following the surgery. The nursing staff were so friendly and empathetic to our situation and would do anything to make our stay as comfortable as possible. We had ladies dropping off toys and blankets, not to mention the Clown Doctors, who would come in and tell a silly joke or make a balloon animal to cheer him up.

The day finally came when we had to take Sam home and begin the next phase of our life. It was all a new experience to us and we would learn as we went along. This was made a bit easier with the help of Vision Australia and we can't thank them enough for preparing us in advance.

Sam adjusted amazingly well and was soon running around the house as if he could see. It's true what they say about kids and their resilience. It would've been a whole lot different if it was one of us that had to go through this experience.

Cleaning out his eye socket after the surgery was heart wrenching. We had to draw strength and courage from Sam and contain our emotions to protect him from the grief we were feeling. It was very difficult looking into a socket where there was once an eye, with nothing in there to look back at you. We made a concerted effort not to be sad or emotional around Sam as we wanted to remain positive and do anything to lift his spirits.

In the early days, I had a lot of trouble accepting Sam's vision impairment. When we would go out in public, I found it hard with the cane, because it felt like it drew a lot of eyes and unwanted attention our way. I didn't want the pity or sorrow from others which I know were with good intentions in mind. To them I was with Sam 'the blind boy' not Sam 'my boy'. I would much rather walk with him hand-in-hand wishing it would all go away and we could get on with our lives as normal. I still find it difficult to park in a disabled car spot, even though we are entitled to.

We were given Sam for a reason. He is here to deliver a message of hope, courage and inspiration to those who have been dealt the wrong cards in life. We all get a hand of cards, but it's how you choose to play with them that's the difference. Life is a blessing, so live it to the fullest.

CHAPTER 1

RETINOBLASTOMA

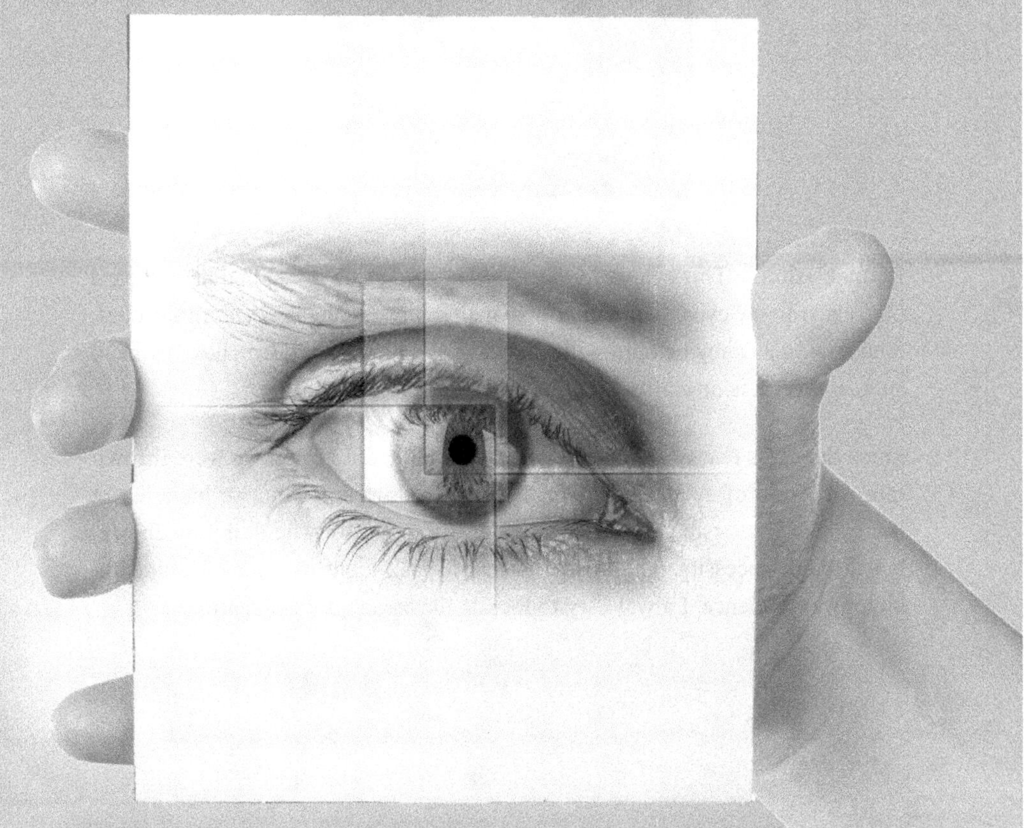

Chapter 1

Retinoblastoma

(Lisa)

Count your blessings and be grateful and thankful for what you have, not what you don't have.

Unknown

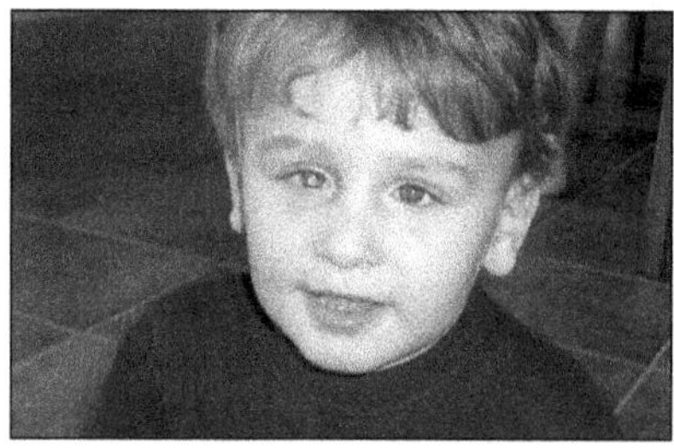

Retinoblastoma. This is a word that, until twelve years ago, I had never heard of. Cancer in the eyes. I didn't know that anybody could get cancer in the eyes. And how can a baby be born with cancer? Even now all of this makes my head spin, and yet it is now all so very clear.

Since Sam was twelve weeks old, whether we liked it or not, we were thrown into the world of eyes and cancer. In the last thirteen years, we have learnt more about these two subjects than we ever thought we would, not by choice, but through necessity. The upside is that it has taught us a lot of incidental biology and science. I always try to look at the upside, free education!

It is thanks to the Ophthalmology and Oncology staff at the Royal Children's Hospital Melbourne who were there to guide us through the minefield that we were thrown into with Sam's diagnosis. They were always there to ask questions of and help out with information. There were no stupid questions, and believe me, I am the person for those. And they would never try to bamboozle us with medical jargon, as so many doctors tend to do.

So now is my chance to explain things for the book. To get an understanding of our journey we went through, to follow I have an explanation of what we were dealing with. I have asked Orthoptist and Retinoblastoma Co-ordinator at the RCH, Sandra Staffieri, to answer some questions for us to be able to explain this nasty little monster we call 'Rb'.

What is retinoblastoma (Rb) and how does it occur in young children?

Retinoblastoma is a rapidly developing cancer that develops from the immature cells of a Retina, the light detecting tissue of the eye. It is the most common malignant tumour of the eye in children.

Retinoblastoma is a rare solid tumour/cancer that develops in one or both eyes of children. Developing cells within the eye keep dividing until the age of about five years, which is why Rb usually stops occurring after this age.

Is it hereditary or sporadic?

The genes in our DNA provide the instructions on how this will occur. Think of DNA as the 'instruction book' for the human body, and each chapter as a gene. Rb is caused by a spelling mistake (gene change) in one chapter of the book – the RB1 gene. This gene is located on a region of the long arm of chromosome 13. This spelling mistake can occur as a new event in an individual (sporadic) or it can be inherited from a parent (hereditary). Each parent contributes half of their chromosomes (and genes) to each child. If a parent has the mutation, there is a 50% chance it will be passed on to each of their children. This would apply for each pregnancy. Genetic testing is available to identify the spelling mistake and provide individuals with choices for management and treatment that are appropriate for them.

In Sam's situation, the gene change in the RB1 gene was sporadic, an accident of Mother Nature as we used to describe it to Sam. They said that at conception, when his cells started to divide, there were two 'hits'. One to cause the gene mutation and the second to develop the tumours.

What are the statistics for Rb?

As a general approximation, the incidence of Rb is 1:15,000–20,000 births. As information was received from the RCH, the following statistics are for Victoria and Tasmania:

In the last 15 years (1997–2010) the incidence is 1:15,000 births.

The previous 15 years (1981–1996) the incidence was 1:17,500

This incidence is on par with the reported literature for the rest of the world.

How many children are diagnosed with either unilateral (one eye) or bilateral (both eyes) Rb each year?

Currently, for Victoria/Tasmania combined between 4–5 new cases are diagnosed each year.

1981–1996: 3.9 new diagnoses per year

1997–2010: 4.6 new diagnoses per year

In the last 15 years, 60% were unilateral and 40% bilateral – this is largely unchanged, although there were more bilateral in the last 15 years compared to previous years.

The number of cases will also depend on the birth rate and if the birth rate increases we could expect to see more cases in line with this. This is clearly demonstrated by considering that 2/3 of the WORLDS cases are in China and India – because their birth rate is so high.

What symptoms should parents be looking for in the early detection of retinoblastoma?

These are the main signs to be aware of:

- *White pupil/abnormal looking coloured PUPIL (Leukocoria) – often noticed in photos. Sometimes called the 'Cat's eye' reflex.*
- *Eye turn – drifting/wandering eye (Strabismus) – often noticed before the white reflex.*
- *There are many other causes for Strabismus and it can occur in about 5% of the population. The presence of Strabismus should always be investigated PROMPTLY to rule out any sinister cause such as retinoblastoma.*
- *Poor vision – this can present as shaking eyes (Nystagmus)*
- *Family history is incredibly important as well. Anyone with a family history of retinoblastoma should see their GP so that a referral can be made to the Clinical Genetics Service in their state for advice and counselling.*

I cannot express how important early detection of this disease is. And to be aware of the signs and be able to recognise them. Looking back in hindsight, we were shown more than one of these signs from very early with Sam, but either didn't recognise them or disregarded them. Although we were lucky to diagnose him at such an early age, who knows if the outcome may have been different if we were able to start treatment earlier.

Sam displayed many of these signs of Rb. He suffered severe Nystagmus. His little eyes would shake back and forth a lot. And today, although his eyes have since been removed, he does still display a slight Nystagmus with his prosthetic eyes.

From very early he was always looking up, towards the sun or a light. We since found out that early on he would have only had vision that gave him a light/dark perception, so he was looking at a light source.

He was never able to focus on anything, including us. That is one thing that upset me as a new mum. When would my baby give me those adoring baby to mum stares and smile at me?

There was a defining moment when we really knew something was wrong. In our two-storey home, Jim was carrying Sam down the stairs one night. Jim told me to have a look at his eyes. In the dim light, his pupils were dilated. We could see lumps in his eyes, milky white looking masses. We now know that we were seeing his tumours.

Also now, looking back at photos of Sam from very young, there is a definite white spot visible in his eyes. When we would first look at the photos, unaware of the problem, we thought it was weird to have a white spot instead of a red spot, but didn't think any more of it.

Oh hindsight, what a wonderful thing you are.

Who should parents contact if they have any questions, concerns or simply require more information about the disease?

There are a number of health professionals that parents can contact as a first port of call if they have any concerns regarding their child showing any of the previously noted signs or symptoms. These would include GP, Maternal Child Health Nurse, Paediatrician or Optometrist. Any one of these individuals should *be able to answer any questions or direct the parent to the right person who can. If this primary health care professional has any concerns they should refer immediately to a Paediatric Ophthalmologist (eye specialist) or call the Ophthalmology (Eye) Department at the Royal Children's Hospital (or equivalent interstate).*

However, in saying this, the first healthcare professional that we brought up our concerns with fobbed us off. "Don't worry, it can take babies up to twelve weeks to focus," he said. Not happy with that, and thankfully trusting our parental intuition, our gut instinct, we brought up our concerns with our Maternal Child Health Nurse, who, after making a few phone calls while we were in her room, pushed to get us an appointment with an Ophthalmologist quickly. My advice to other parents who may know that something is wrong but can't quite pinpoint what it is, or has a health professional say something they are not completely happy with – keep pushing. It is your parental right to question the 'health professionals'. To them it's a job, to you it's your child's life.

What type of treatments and options are available for newly diagnosed children?

Treatment for retinoblastoma depends on a number of factors:

Age of child, one or both eyes involved, number of tumours, size of tumours, position in the eye of the tumours, whether there has been disease spread outside of the eye.

Each child is evaluated for all of these and the best treatment options are offered to the family. This can include any one or more of the following:

Chemotherapy, cryotherapy (freezing the tumour), laser therapy (heating the tumour), radiation therapy, brachytherapy (radioactive plaque), intra-arterial or intra-vitreal chemotherapy (chemotherapy directly to the eye).

The most common treatment for smaller tumours is chemotherapy combined with laser therapy.

The most common surgical treatment for very advanced disease is removal of the eye – enucleation.

Sam has had every one of these treatments, once or numerous times. We hit his eyes with every possible form of attack that we could. In some ways, I wish that we hadn't inflicted so much upon his tiny body, knowing now what the eventual outcome was. But we can always hold our heads high and know that we did absolutely everything that we could do to try to save his life and his sight.

The first plan of attack was chemotherapy. That was really hard to see – a three-month-old baby hooked up to an IV, knowing it was pumping poison into him to try to kill this enemy. The bonus of the chemo was that it shrunk his tumours in his right eye enough for his retina in the eye to partly reattach. That gave him a little bit of useable vision in that eye. He only had peripheral vision, no central vision, but it was enough to show him a bit of the world and learn things like colours and shapes, vision which would stay with him until he lost that eye over four years later.

When Sam would go into the RCH for an EUA (examination under anaesthetic), usually on a monthly basis, he would more often than not have some localised therapy administered. This would be either laser therapy or cryotherapy. Laser therapy was ok, he would come out of the treatment generally happy and not in pain. Cryotherapy, however, a whole different story. This was when Sam would have liquid nitrogen placed on the surface of the eye, or the eye would be cut and the liquid nitrogen put into the eye. He would come out from theatre looking like he'd done ten rounds with a prize fighter. His face around his eyes would be swollen and develop bruising and he wouldn't be able to open his eyes for days. But I think that the worst part was the two weeks of follow up eye drops, two different drops, four times a day each. We would literally have to pin him on the floor, usually taking more than just one of us. We would then have to pry his incredibly sore eyes open to apply the drops. This would usually end with more than one of us crying. I hated that part.

Sam had radiation therapy, at Peter MacCallum Cancer Institute in Melbourne. It was a full routine we got into, five days a week for four weeks. We would fast him from midnight, drive in peak hour traffic into the city, put him under anaesthetic, be fitted into his specially moulded and fitted face mask to keep him in position, have five minutes of treatment, wake him up in recovery, then go home, to do it all again the next day. We would be home by 10:30 am, ready to restart the day.

He had three radioactive plaques implanted, about a year apart from each other. This was at The Royal Victorian Eye and Ear Hospital. In to theatre to have his eye cut open, and a radioactive piece of metal implanted. This would stay in his eye for about two days while he was an in-patient, then was surgically removed. The first one that he had implanted caused him the most pain and discomfort that I had ever seen him go through. The nurses would try to tell me to keep at least a one metre distance from him as he was 'radioactive', but tell that to a miserable two-year-old who just wants comfort from his mummy. That rule didn't last long at all.

The second one he had implanted was hard for me, as I was pregnant with Mitchell. I was not allowed to be in the hospital with him. Jim stayed with him, with me at home. Knowing what pain he was experiencing was painful for me, that I couldn't be there to hold him.

Our final effort was the chemo injection directly into his right eye, done under anaesthetic. In the end, it didn't work, but we had to try.

This all lead up to the final surgeries, enucleation. What an awful word. I hate it so much. Surprisingly, being the most final and devastating of surgeries, it was the surgery or treatment that caused him some of the least amount of pain, but caused us the most amount of emotional pain. Taking him into surgery the day of the second eye being removed was the worst time of our lives. The anaesthetist said that only one of us could be in there when he drifted off to sleep thanks to the 'chocolate mask'. "This is the last time that he will ever see us, we are both staying," I said. Take that Mr Gas Man!

Are there regular examinations at the hospital to monitor the disease?

Under five years of age, where necessary, the examinations are conducted whilst the child is under general anaesthetic. For many children in the first few years, this could almost be every month.

This is so that the eye can be adequately examined for any new tumours, which if treated early will have less impact on their vision. Once the child is over five years, awake examinations are possible.

How long does treatment usually last and what is the follow up procedure?

Duration of treatment will depend on the size of tumours, eyes affected and what treatment is undertaken. The older the child becomes, the less often they will need to be reviewed. For those children that have had an eye removed, this is to make sure the prosthetic (artificial) eye is fitting well, and no other type of eye disease occurs in their only good eye. Children with only one eye affected and proven to not have heritable Rb will be examined periodically into early adulthood. Children with bilateral disease, have a somewhat longer course of treatment until they turn five years of age. Then they will be examined every six months/yearly to ensure they are managing with the residual vision they have in their remaining eye. Children with both eyes affected, and a small percentage of children with one eye affected, are at a higher risk of developing second cancers in their lifetime. They will have ongoing follow up with specialist doctors for their lifetime.

Maintaining contact with Rb families is also important so that when they have children, they know to be examined early.

What is the success rate for remission with the early diagnosis of the disease? How many children lose one or both eyes from the condition?

Rb can respond differently in different individuals. New tumours can develop up until the age of five years, but this slows down fairly rapidly once the child reaches the age of one. Tumours may remain inactive for a while, but then 'fire up' again at any point in the first five years when the retinal cells are still developing.

Currently, most children with only one affected eye, lose the affected eye. This is because it presents too late for any other treatment as the tumour is too big and the risk of it spreading outside the eye is too great. Rb is a very aggressive cancer once it spreads out of the eye.

Children with both eyes affected, usually have one less affected eye, and this is the one that is saved. The vision that they retain will depend on the position of the tumours and the type of treatment they need to stop its progression.

Sam had bilateral Rb, tumours in both eyes. As detailed above, the tumours in his right eye were inactive for over a year while treatment continued on his left eye. After removing his left eye, the tumours in the right eye 'fired up' again. These tumours in the end could not be controlled, and the decision was made that the risk of the cancer spreading from the eye was too great. I don't say that the doctors made him blind, but that they saved his life.

What are the possibilities of future secondary cancers/tumours and is this caused by the disease and/or treatment?

Children or adult survivors who have a germ line RB1 mutation are at increased risk of developing secondary cancers – not associated with the eye. Avoidance of smoking and sun exposure can reduce the risk for lung and skin cancers. In some instances, previous radiation treatment for the eye in childhood can increase the risk of tumours in the area of the radiation 'in-field'. This is particularly true for sarcomas of the bony socket of the eye.

I've said it before; I'll say it again. Cancer – the gift that keeps on giving.

The fact that he has had cancer increases his risks of secondary cancer. And the treatment that he had to save his life could also be the cause of secondary cancer. You have to weigh up the risk of non-treatment versus future risk of having had treatment.

As a parent of a child who has been through such a 'this won't happen to us' situation, I now have trouble not being paranoid and jumping to conclusions when Sam is sick. I have to realise that a simple cold is not pneumonia, a bruise on his leg does not mean leukaemia, and a headache does not mean a brain tumour. I am still yet to find out when this paranoia will end. Or will it ever?

What happens if families want to have more children? Is there any way that the parents can be tested or is there anything that can prevent this from reoccurring?

Genetic testing and counselling is a very important part of caring for families and their children with Rb.

Each state in Australia has a genetic counselling service, and would be able to provide appropriate and relevant advice for each individual or family, depending on the clinical and genetic information that is available.

If the RB1 gene is identified for a family, there are a number of different prenatal (before birth) tests available to determine if the baby also has the gene change. Pre-natal diagnosis (PND) may be used very early in the pregnancy to determine whether the baby has the RB1 mutation. This assists the doctors' planning for the arrival of, and screening for tumours in a baby who may likely develop Rb. The earliest possible detection of the tumours may influence the treatments available and possibly afford a better outcome with regards to maximising the child's vision or retaining their eye. Genetic testing, either before or after a baby is born can also eliminate the need for multiple eye examinations under general anaesthetic if the baby is found not to carry their family's RB1 mutation.

If the RB1 gene is known some couples may decide to use assisted reproductive technologies such, as IVF and, pre-implantation diagnosis (PGD) to select an embryo that does not carry the RB1 mutation. For some families, this may not be the option of choice.

In some cases, the RB1 gene change cannot be identified through testing. However, it is important that doctors are aware of the family history of retinoblastoma so that the couple and their doctor can make appropriate decisions regarding screening and management for their child.

It is important to remember, however, that the choices individuals make are very personal, and can be a very sensitive matter. Each parent will make a choice that is right for them.

We had our genetic testing completed before we tried to fall pregnant with our next child, Mitchell. I have always said that if we would have to go through it again as parents, we would. But I don't think that I could have willingly put another child through what Sam went through.

Our genetics came back clear for Jim and I, but showed that Sam now has the RB1 gene mutation. Despite this clearing Jim and I, Mitchell and Caitlin were still tested by the Ophthalmologists at the RCH at about two weeks old and genetically tested through blood taken at or soon after birth.

Can the children that have retinoblastoma pass this gene/condition on to their offspring? What are the percentages?

Only children with a germ line mutation (gene change that is present in every cell of their body) can pass it on to their children. All children with both eyes affected will have a germ line mutation. It is possible however, for an individual to have one eye affected and still have a germ line mutation. Germ line mutations are found in approximately 30% of affected individuals. Of these, around 25% inherited this gene change from a parent. If a child is shown to have a germ line mutation, with each pregnancy there is a 50% chance that this gene change will be passed on to their children. Sometimes, but not very often, an individual can have the RB1 mutation but not develop the disease. We don't really understand why, but this is subject to current research. Our understanding of how this happens will be useful for future treatments to be developed, such as gene therapy.

Can parents contact other families to discuss their experiences and get an insight into what to expect?

In Victoria, the Retinoblastoma Care Co-ordinator can put families in touch with each other for support at any time during or after their child's treatment. Many families are very happy to be a support to newly diagnosed families or individuals who had Rb and are planning to have children. This opportunity is vital to each family's coping strategies with disease, and seeing that there is light at the end of the tunnel. They can also seek professional support through their care team.

We found this support group of families essential in helping us get through this ordeal. They could tell us that they knew how we were feeling, and they really did. They had been through, or were still going through what we were. We would also meet up with a lot of the families at the EUAs. One Wednesday every month was 'Eye Day' at the RCH Day Surgery Department. They would have a theatre list for all of the children with Rb, or those who had a family history of Rb to get checked or treated while under anaesthetic. I found this an invaluable informal support, while we would spend hours in the waiting room for our children to go into theatre. We are still friends with some of these families today. You know who you are. We would not have survived without you. Thank you.

There are also many other sources of help, support and information that we have come across through this wild ride. Some contacts we were offered, some we had to ask about, and others we simply stumbled across. We found during the process that it was sometimes only when we asked about information or support that we were offered it. When you don't know what questions to ask it makes it difficult. We have listed as many resources in our resource section that we could think of, even some that would have been useful to us thirteen years ago if we had have known.

CHAPTER 2

GRIEF

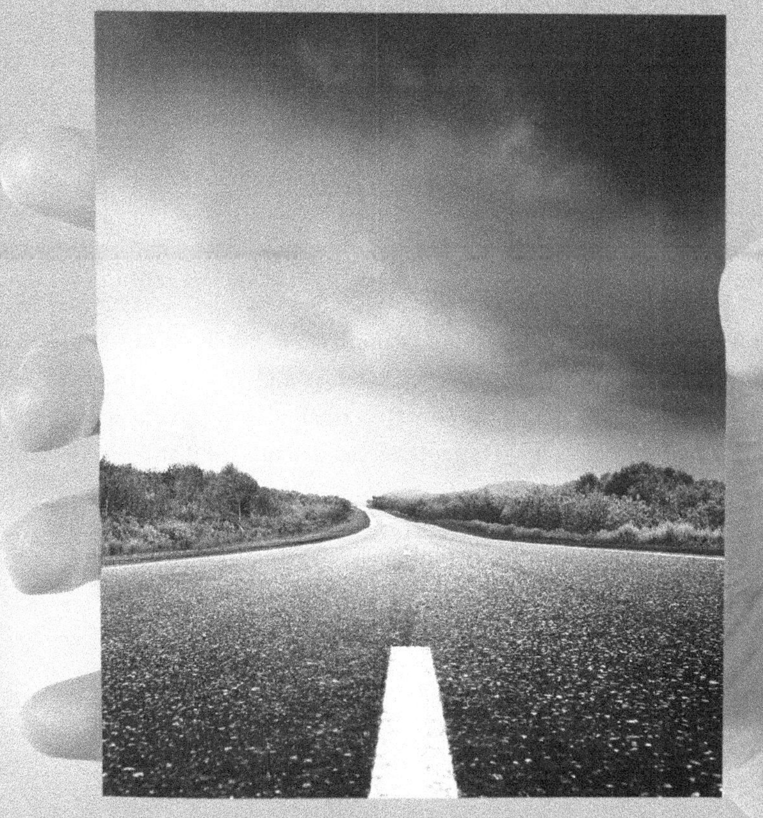

Chapter 2

Grief

(Lisa)

Don't play the 'What If?' game,
because you're never going to win

'All Saints' Cast Member
Seven Network Australia

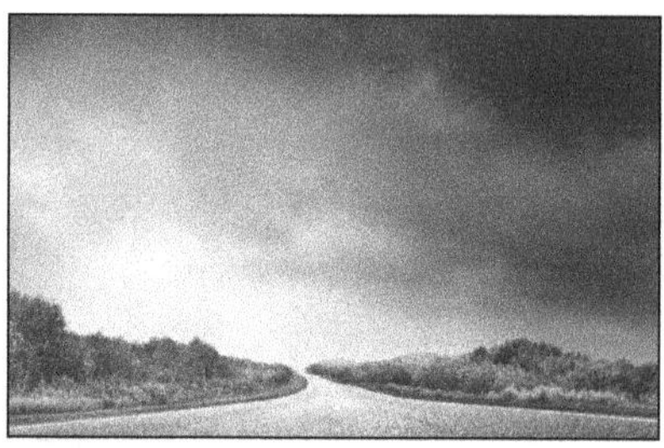

Grief. Well, well, well. Where do I start?

Grief has played such a major role in this adventure of ours. It has affected all of us in many different ways, at many different times and for varied lengths of time. And I know that it will continue to affect us all at the different stages of Sam's life in the future. Good old retinoblastoma, it's the gift that keeps on giving!

According to 'Dictionary.com', the definition of grief is "1. Keen mental suffering or distress over affliction or loss; sharp sorrow; painful regret. 2. A cause or occasion of keen distress or sorrow".

I like the definition of grief from the Victorian Government Better Health website: "Grief is a normal, natural and inevitable response to loss. It can affect every part of our life, including our thoughts, feelings, behaviours, beliefs, physical health and our relationships with others. Grief does not have a timeline and can be felt over an extended period of time. With the support of family and friends, most people gradually find ways to learn to live with loss... Many people experience feelings of sadness, anger, anxiety, fear and numbness... Grief is a process, not an event. It is a journey, not a destination."

It used to be believed that there were various stages of grief. These included such emotions as denial, anger, bargaining and acceptance. Grief actually includes a wide range of emotions, thoughts and behaviours. Everybody moves through grief in their own way, grief doesn't always happen in a predictable and orderly way. Even when we seem to be getting on with life, the reality is that most of us will continue to grieve in subtle ways for the rest of our lives.

Everybody experiences grief differently. A person's experience of grief is influenced by many factors.

These can include:

- The age of the person (child, adolescent or adult)
- Religious or spiritual beliefs
- Cultural practices
- Availability of support from family, friends and community
- Associated stresses (e.g. relationship breakdown, job loss, financial difficulties)

Grief includes a wide range of emotions, thoughts and behaviours. People may experience some or all of many reactions associated with grief. Some of the many reactions, but not all of them may include:

- Anger
- Anxiety
- Panic
- Change in world view
- Change in values and beliefs
- Confusion
- Sadness
- Numbness
- Depression
- Sleeping difficulties
- Physical symptoms
- Changes in appetite
- Low self-esteem
- Difficulty concentrating
- Inability to cope
- Guilt or remorse
- Helplessness
- Hopelessness
- Loneliness
- Relief
- Shock and disbelief

As stated in the definition of grief, it is related to a 'loss'. What loss did we suffer, our beautiful boy is still alive? But we have suffered many 'losses' from when Sam was diagnosed, and I believe that we all will keep suffering these losses for the rest of his life.

Our beautiful first born baby boy was diagnosed with cancer. We were told he had a life-threatening illness that would also threaten any possibility of him having 'normal' vision. The first specialist that we saw told us, very matter-of-factly, "His retinas are detached. There's only a slight chance that he'll ever see. And if it is cancer, both eyes have to be removed." With those couple of sentences spoken calmly from her, it felt like our hearts were ripped from our chests and then set on fire.

Two days later, when Sam was officially diagnosed at the Royal Children's Hospital Melbourne, our heads were spinning when they told us the results of the tests. What did this mean for our son, who we thought had his entire life ahead of him? Would he survive through cancer? Would he ever see? What did the future hold for him? It was there that we encountered our first feelings of loss. The plans, hopes and dreams that we had for our beautiful son, whose life had only just begun, were all destroyed that day. We have since learned that while we thought that these had been torn away from the three of us, we just needed to make new and different plans. I was talking to Sam about this the other day, the need for flexibility. I was telling him that while your ideas and plans may not always work out how you want, and it is sometimes about having the flexibility to make new plans or dreams.

Although it is now nine years since the removal of Sam's second eye, and he has been cleared of cancer, the grief for all of us continues. And as I stated earlier, I'm sure it will continue for the rest of Sam's life, in some way, large or small. We have grieved and will continue to grieve over many issues of the whole cancer and vision loss journey. The grief of the cancer diagnosis, watching him suffer through the treatments, the loss of his eyes, learning to be a blind person in a very visual world. And then moving forward into the future, not so much living with the grief, but fear of the possibilities. The opportunities (or lack of) available to Sam, will he marry and have children of his own, will his children be condemned to the same fate as him, will he have his dream career, and the list goes on.

I already feel grief with two specific aspects of his future. Firstly, how will he feel when he is eighteen and all of his friends are getting their driver's licences? Secondly, at the moment, Sam's dream career is to be an anaesthetist. Would you use a blind anaesthetist for a surgery? But I have to realise that this is my grief, for something that may never be an issue for him. He may and probably will change his career choice between childhood and adulthood. The licence issue, Sam is already talking about the 'Google Car', something that may well be easily accessible when it is time for him to get his licence.

Jim and I have always dealt with our grief in very different ways and at different times.

Ladies first…

Soon after Sam was born, I knew something was wrong, but I couldn't pinpoint what it was. Call it mother's intuition. Being my firstborn, with a traumatic birth, lack of sleep, unsettled baby (looking back, knowing now it was probably due to not being able to see, perhaps feeling unwell) and all the other fun stuff that new mums go through, I think that I was on the brink of post-natal depression. I remember as soon as they diagnosed him, I said in the hospital recovery room "Well if I didn't have post-natal depression before, I definitely do now!" My first reaction was feeling like I was going to vomit, I felt physically sick.

Once I got over the initial feelings of shock and loss, I think that I handled my grief amazingly well. We were quickly thrown into the cancer process. Within ten days of diagnosis, Sam was starting his first round of chemotherapy. Everything steamrolled from there, with no time for grief. I found that I was just going through the motions, keeping to the schedule of treatments, EUAs (examination under anaesthetic), and a new 'normal' childhood for Sam.

When people would ask me what was happening with Sam, I would calmly talk to them about him, what was going on with his progress. I would tell people about the condition, treatment and possible outcomes. I would talk to people in a clinical 'matter-of-fact' way. Looking back, I see it as being disconnected, that way I could talk about it without getting emotional. It was my way of coping with what was happening. It was my therapy. I would talk openly and honestly to everybody about how I was 'feeling'. People would say they couldn't believe how well I was handling it. "I couldn't do it" they would say. My response was, “I’m his mum, I have no choice”. It was when I would stop and listen to the words that I was saying and think about it that I would get upset.

It was only after Sam had his second eye removed that I really fell apart. No more hospital, no more monthly anaesthetics, lots of time to think. Never a good thing for me. I was preoccupied previously, now I had all of the built up thoughts running through my head. “What have we just done?” I would look back over the time since diagnosis, think of all of the pain we had put him through, all of his childhood that was lost. The mother guilt would come up. I would ask myself what kind of mother I was to give my son cancer. I knew that it was just ‘one of those things’ – ‘an accident of Mother Nature’ as everybody would say. But on my bad days, I felt responsible. Sometimes, even occasionally now, more than nine years later, I can get very upset about all that has happened.

A year before Sam’s second eye was removed, I gave birth to our cheeky bundle Mitchell. Soon after that, I decided I needed to do something about what I was going through. I found that my good days were good, but my bad days were like I had plummeted into an abyss. I needed to get a balance. I was having counselling through Vision Australia and decided it was time to put my hand up for help, bite the bullet and start on medication for depression. I knew that I needed to be there for Sam, Mitchell and Jim, and that I could only do that with help.

I still fight with depression today and I will do so I think for a while. One of the not-so-wonderful by-products of grief, yet an entity all of its own. Again an issue that different people go through so differently.

By definition, as per the Beyond Blue website, “Depression is more than a low mood – it’s a serious illness that has an impact on both physical and mental health. While we all feel sad, moody or low from time to time, some people experience these feelings intensely, for long periods of time (weeks, months or even years) and sometimes without any apparent reason.”

Jim, on the other hand, is a whole different story.

We were both in shock over the original diagnosis. But what I remember most from that day of diagnosis at the hospital was Jim's statement. We were told that if Sam had retinoblastoma, the doctors would also do a lumbar puncture while he was under anaesthetic to see if the cancer had spread. They said that if he had this procedure, he would have a band aid on his back. We were sitting in the recovery room with our tiny baby in our arms. Jim pulled up Sam's top and looked at his back… band aid. Jim looked up. "That's just killed me!" Sam had cancer. Our worst fears were confirmed.

Jim dealt with grief in the early days very differently to how I did. He buried his grief down, shutting the world out. He didn't speak to people about what was going on and how he was feeling about it. He lost touch and connection with a lot of friends. It was easier not to see people than to see them and have to explain what was going on.

Jim also went through a lot of anger with his grief. If we were to take Sam out as a young baby or toddler, he would look at other 'normal' kids. Why were they able to do things that our son would possibly never be able to do? It wasn't fair that they were able to enjoy life when Sam couldn't.

The time that I noticed this the most was when Mitchell was born. Seeing Jim's reaction to our beautiful second son was not one that a father should have. Looking in retrospect, he was angry that Mitchell was the 'perfect son' that Sam should have been. Why should Mitchell be able to do things that his older brother can't? Early on, I actually felt worried about leaving Mitchell alone with Jim. How ridiculous, that a mother can't leave her son with his own father. But I was afraid that something might 'happen'. Not that anything would, Jim is the most loving father my kids could have. But I was.

Jim suffered silently with his grief for a very long time in his own way. I would suggest that he see somebody, talk to somebody, consider medication as an option. "I'm fine," would be the answer that I would always get back.

It has only been through the writing of this book that I have finally seen Jim really dealing with his grief and depression. I have seen a massive transformation in him. I am a lot less worried about him than I have been for a long, long time.

The way that Jim and I handled our grief was very different. Through a lot of our journey, I felt like we were two trains, running side by side on two tracks, yet travelling separately. We were there for each other, but not really. But, in saying that, it must have been what we both needed and could cope with at that time. Unfortunately, we met couples going through the same situation with their children at hospital whose relationships or marriages didn't survive. More than just simply surviving through Sam's sickness, Jim and I as a couple have become stronger together.

One thing that we have both learnt to do, together or separately, is to not hide our grief or feelings from Sam. A wise person once told us that it is ok to show Sam that we are upset or sad about what is happening and how we feel about it. I remember sitting with him shortly before his operation to remove his second eye. I was telling this four-and-a-half-year-old, very wise beyond his young years, how he was going to have the operation that would make him blind. "Mummy and Daddy are really sad and upset about it. You won't be able to see when you wake up in the hospital bed. It's going to be hard, but we are here to help each other. And if we all need to cry and be sad about it, that's ok."

We have always talked to Sam about how we were feeling and how he is feeling. Not so often now, but in the past he and I would talk about how we were feeling. He would quite often say to me, soon after he became blind, "I hate that I can't see Mummy, I wish that the doctors could make me see again." But now he will follow that up with "…But if I wasn't blind, I couldn't do Braille, and I like doing Braille."

Sam has also been a very big player in the grieving process. After all, it is our child, but it is the rest of his life. When he was diagnosed, and the years of treatment that followed, it was the 'easy' time for him. Sounds stupid to say that, but doing the hospital thing from three months old, he did not know that life was meant to be any different. Although hospital more often than not meant treatment and pain, we used to say that he looked at the hospital as if it was his own 'Luna Park'. He would look forward to when the next trip into the RCH would be. "When am I having my next chocolate mask?" he would ask. This would refer to the anaesthetic, when the anaesthetists would put chocolate flavouring (essence) in the mask to detract from the smell of the anaesthetic gas. He got used to these, having well over one hundred anaesthetics in his young life.

It has only really been in the last few years that the grief for Sam has set in for him. We are having a hard time, especially now. Sam has a lot of things on his plate. He is in Year 8 at high school. He is also starting to head into puberty. These are both things that regular teenagers have to deal with. But Sam must deal with a number of other factors as well.

Sam is super-intelligent, I say as all proud mums do of their kids. But he is very switched on, both intellectually and of what is happening around him. He is realising that the gap between himself and the other boys at school is getting bigger. The other boys are getting more into sports, computers and video games, and generally 'hanging out' with their friends. These are 'normal' boy activities that parents would take for granted, that we know are more difficult or not achievable for Sam.

Another big problem at the moment is that his younger brother, Mitchell, is passing him in a lot of his own actions, activities and achievements. Sam is showing a lot of anger and resentment towards him for this.

Over the last couple of years, we have seriously looked into the social and behavioural side of Sam. He had been portraying physical, verbal and emotional anger, obsessive compulsive traits (symptoms of OCD), and not coping with situations that didn't go to his plans or were out of routine for him. After discussion with the RCH Long Term Follow Up team, we even had him assessed to see if he was on the autism spectrum, which he was not. After looking further into the situation with psychologists, the answers put forward to us seemed to make everything clear.

They explained to us that we are dealing with a young child who has had to deal with an amazingly grown-up traumatic experience. Life has dealt him a hand that many adults would not cope with, let alone a child. He has not coped with what has happened. The psychologist explained 'Inside Outside' feelings to us. Inside he is feeling vulnerable, frustrated, nervous, anxious and scared, but he brings out these feelings as anger, aggression and resentment.

Dealing with Sam's grief is in many ways more challenging than dealing with his blindness. It is hard enough to cope with our own grief, but even harder to help Sam cope with his. As a parent, you just want to be able to put a band aid on your child's 'ouch' to make the pain go away. This 'ouch' is so much harder to fix.

The one bonus about Sam's attitude is that he is very strong-willed and stubborn. I always say that these traits are hard to deal with in a thirteen-year-old, but will get him far in life as a blind adult. I can imagine as an adult people will tell him he can't do something, and I know that his response will be "Watch Me!" I hope that Sam will learn to be the kind of person that can look at any challenge that faces him and see the positive in it.

I learnt a long time ago that being angry or upset about a negative situation is not going to change it. Being angry at the world about his cancer and disability wasn't going to make it go away and let him see again. He is blind, but he is here.

CHAPTER 3

DEALING WITH GRIEF

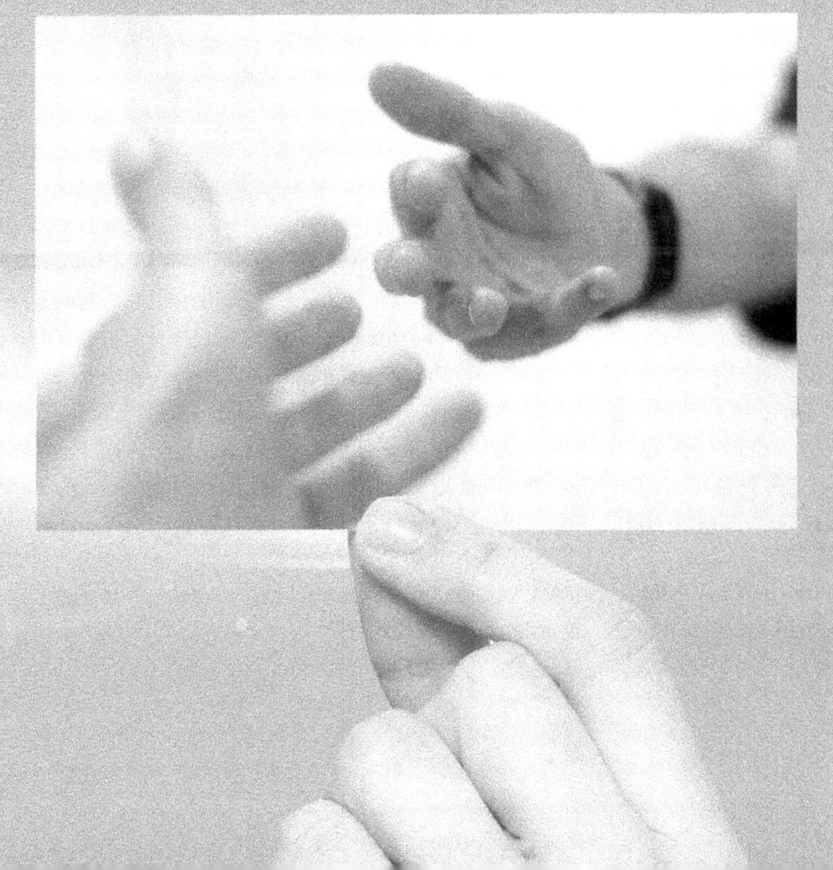

Chapter 3

Dealing with Grief

(Lisa)

Scars only show us where we've been,
they do not dictate where we are going.

Unknown

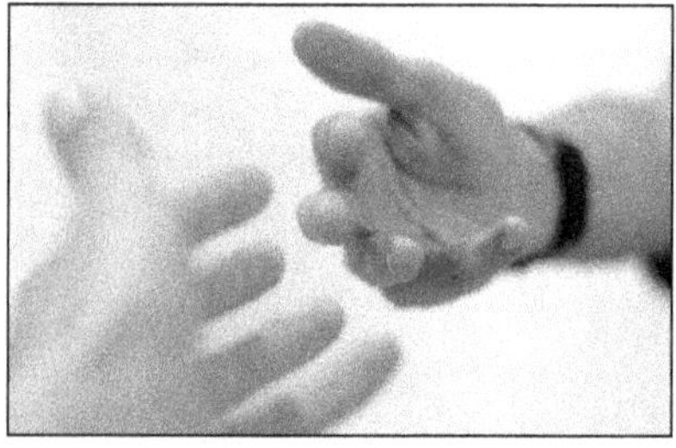

As I stated in the previous chapter about grief, influenced by many factors, people experience different reactions associated to grief.

At many points along this rollercoaster journey of ours, I have wondered if I would ever be able to cope with my grief and get out of the dark abyss that I was in. There have been many times when my head would be spinning, I have felt like I couldn't breathe, like I would vomit, I couldn't control my emotions, have not been able to stop crying. There have been many times when I thought that there was no hope and I've not known what I can do to make things any better.

To this day I still feel grief. My version of grief comes out as depression more so than other reactions towards the situation. Being a first time mum with

Sam, and also going through other tough pregnancies and births at a time of uncertainty for Sam and our family, I also believe that I suffered from post-natal depression.

I know that there is no way I would have survived then, and still now, without the support, friendship and love of those around me. My first coping mechanism was to talk to those closest to me. I was able to talk openly and honestly about what we were going through with Sam. Family and friends were my first port of call and always there when I needed them, especially my Mum and Dad. No matter how much grief they were going through as grandparents, they were always there for me, putting their feelings aside for Jim, Sam and I.

But I found that I also needed to seek professional help, through the counselling services of Vision Australia. I remember calling a phone number for Vision Australia that I found in the phonebook, the day after Sam was diagnosed. The poor lady who happened to answer the phone to me, Sandy, had to deal with a devastated mother on the other end. "My baby is going to be blind" I blurted out to her, then burst into tears. Making that call was one of the best things that I have ever done. From then on I had Vision Australia as part of our 'team', helping us in so many ways, even still today and for years to come. But I think what I have felt most helpful from Vision Australia is the emotional support that I have received along the way.

The Vision Australia counselling was definitely something that I couldn't have done without. The time I needed it most I found was when I was pregnant with Mitchell, with the regular fears that any expectant mother has, plus a bigger worry that Mitchell would also be born with Rb. Counselling continued also after he was born and up to and shortly after Sam lost his second eye. The best aspect that I found with the counselling was that I could just talk about how I was feeling, verbalise my emotions. The counsellor didn't need to respond or offer any solutions or give me advice, unlike what family might feel they needed to do. Just the fact that I would get it all out was what I needed to do.

I accepted that I needed to do something more about my depression when I found out I was pregnant with Mitchell. Very soon after Mitchell was born I started on anti-depressants. The biggest problem I had with that was that I felt like I was giving in, that I would have been judged by those around me for resorting to drugs. But I found support in my decision from the medical people supporting me. They explained that it wouldn't blur my consciousness and make me like an unemotional zombie, but take the edge off my extremes of emotions so that I could have a little more clarity. It definitely benefitted me and something that I probably would have been a lot worse without.

I also joke that during the hard times, my Psychologist's name was 'Dr Cadbury'. Chocolate got me through a lot of hard times, and there was nothing wrong with that.

These are the methods of coping with grief and depression that I found most helpful for me personally. However, everybody is different. Jim coped, or didn't, very differently to me. He withdrew from those around him, choosing not to have to talk about what was going on and how he was feeling.

Looking at grief and all the feelings, reactions and emotions that go along with it, I realise that there are many different ways of coping, and different people will find some methods more useful than others. But where do you start? I think with whatever feels best for you.

Also when different situations that cause grief come up, at different stages and times in your life, how you react to them and cope with them will possibly be different. While we were writing this book, my Mum passed away from lung cancer. How I am dealing with that now is not the same as how I dealt with my grief throughout Sam's journey.

Here are some coping strategies that I have come across throughout my journey.

Acknowledge there is a problem

This is HUGE, well I think so. Possibly the worst thing that I could have done would have been to try to deny there was something wrong and that I could battle on through like everything was ok. Not dealing with grief makes it harder to cope with other stresses that may come later. Give yourself permission to grieve.

Cry

Crying is great, I'm a big fan of this. And I have not been afraid to show my emotions in front of others. Trying to supress emotions can do all sorts of damage. And we have never hidden our emotions from Sam. We needed to let him know that what was happening to him was upsetting us also. It may be helpful to have a regular time and place to allow yourself to be sad.

Time alone

Some people find this helpful. I grew up as an only child, so got used to being my own company from a very early age. I quite often feel the need to 'get away' from those around me to clear my head. Jim would say it wouldn't take long!

Talking to others

People find comfort in having others around them, people with whom they can be sad. The company of others can be comforting, especially if these people have some similar experiences and understanding. We found talking to other families of Rb or blind kids incredibly supportive. They say that they understood what we were going through, and they really did.

Friends and family

Time with family and friends is essential. It is wonderful to be able to share your experiences with those closest to you, but also to be able to be involved in 'normal' experiences and discussions, not related to the source of the grief. Distraction is a wonderful thing.

Support team

Surround yourself with a 'support team'. This is not the time to have 'toxic' people around you. The people who are there for support should be understanding, be a good listener and not be afraid to share their emotions. They should have a clear sense of boundaries and ethics, to be able to resist the temptation to impose their beliefs or tell you how to feel. These support people can be family, friends, colleagues, neighbours, or professional support such as doctors, counsellors and psychologists.

Professional help and support

Both Jim and I have learnt that it is not weak to put up your hand and ask for help. I felt stronger to admit that I needed professional help and to know that it was out there for me. Jim did try a little bit of counselling, but found it not right for him at the time. I was so proud of him to at least give it a try. Depending on the individual, there are different options available for professional help. There are anonymous 'Helplines', the family doctor, counsellors, social workers, psychologists, psychiatrists, ministers and priests and other community groups, support groups with families in a similar situation. We have included a list of professional support services in the Resource Section at the back of the book.

Looking after yourself

This is something that I'm guessing most people going through grief would put on the back-burner, but it is absolutely essential to survive the ordeal. When Sam was first diagnosed, I was so concerned about him and his health that I would forget about me. To be there for Sam and others, I kept being reminded that I needed to look after myself. Isn't that what they tell you in a flight emergency on a plane, put your oxygen mask on before you help others with theirs?

There are many areas of your body and life that need to be looked after during times of grief, and below are some ways in which this can be achieved.

- Diet. Although my first line of defence to cope with stress and grief is always to reach for the chocolate (not that there is anything wrong with that), you need to be fuelling your body with the right things. Grief can lead to a loss of appetite and tastes may change. Rather than trying to eat a full meal, grazing on healthy foods may be better, such as fruit vegetables, yoghurt, cereal, soup and salads. Although it may seem comforting, it's best to avoid spicy, fatty food or junk food, which can be hard to digest. Vitamins may also help a lot during these times, for the body to get a healthy balance of what is needed.

- Exercise and activity. What's better than getting some fresh air and sunshine when you're not feeling quite right?

- Pampering and nurturing.

- Relaxation and sleep.

- Care with addictive substances.

- Do something you love.

- Write a diary or journal.

- Music.

- Retail therapy – a personal favourite.

Some people may find my list of suggestions above useful, some may have their own ideas of ways to nurture themselves. There are no hard and fast rules, as long as you are looking after YOU.

Know that you can come through this. You may never be the same person again, but you can survive this.

CHAPTER 4

MALE DEPRESSION

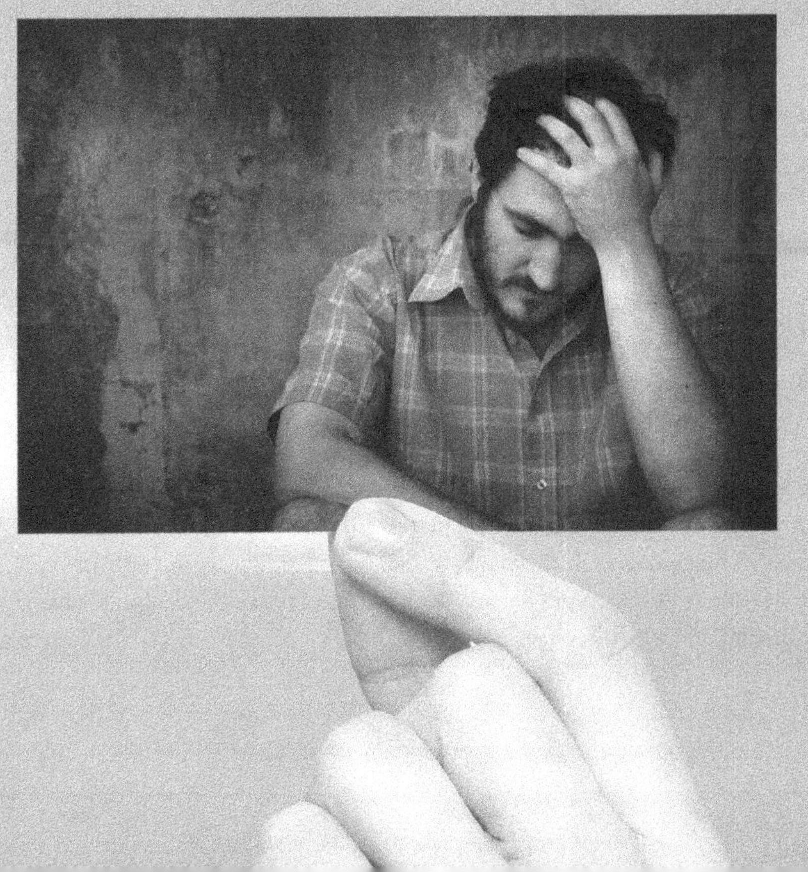

Chapter 4

Male Depression

(Jim)

Depression is the inability to construct a future.

Rollo May

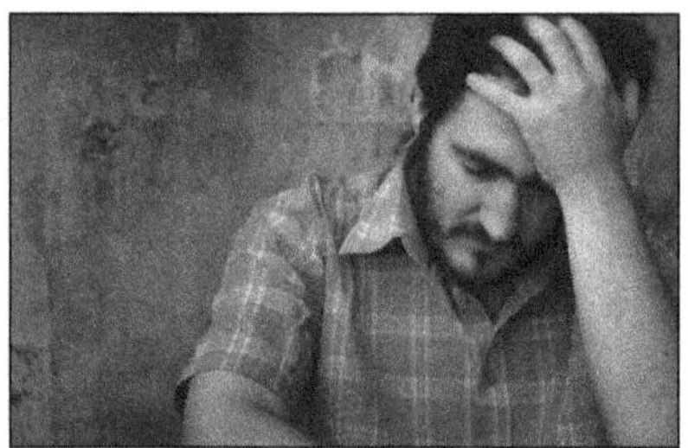

It was something that Winston Churchill described as his 'black dog', but for me it was more like a black cloud that hovered over my head wherever I went, from the moment I woke up to the time I went to sleep. Depression is a debilitating disease that can affect you in every aspect of your life, mentally, physically and emotionally and it is quite often overlooked as a bout of sadness or unhappiness. Lisa explained it to me like she was in an 'Abyss', a big black hole.

We can all experience a range of emotions when something bad happens in our life and more often than not this mood will pass after a few hours or days. However, for some people this mood of feeling sad or low doesn't go away and can develop into something deeper, such as a depressive disorder and have a significant effect on their lives.

At my lowest point I didn't want to leave the house other than to go to work, of which I had no choice. Besides the hospital, our house was a safe haven for me where I could hide and I didn't have to tell anyone how I was feeling. I totally withdrew from socialising, exercising or participating in life because it was much easier. I felt extreme guilt about experiencing anything that was fun and joyous, because after all why should I be happy when Sam was going through such a difficult time. I remember consciously stopping myself from laughing and smiling. It took me a long time to break out of this way of thinking. I was just going through the motions and merely existing, doing what I had to do to keep the family unit going financially.

If you have been feeling this way every day for at least two weeks and have many of the following symptoms, then I would strongly suggest speaking to a professional or contacting an organisation that can give you some clarity and options on the next course of action.

Some symptoms may include…

- an unusually sad mood
- a loss of enjoyment or interest in activities you used to enjoy
- lack of energy and tiredness
- feeling worthless or guilty when you are not really at fault
- thinking about death a lot
- having difficulty concentrating or making decisions
- moving more slowly than usual
- becoming agitated
- having sleeping difficulties or sleeping too much
- a change in eating habits such as loss of appetite or eating too much

Every person will differ in the number of symptoms they have and also the severity.

There are some great organisations out there that can assist you and point you in the right direction, such as Beyond Blue, Black Dog Institute, Life Line and MensLine, to name a few. Even if you think you're OK and you can't admit to yourself that you may have depression, there are tests and questionnaires that you can do online to help you identify the symptoms, such as the Kessler Psychological Distress Scale (K10), Diagnostic and Statistical Manual (DSM), Sphere Questionnaire and The Burns Depression Checklist.

There has been a stigma attached to mental health, particularly for men. I'm not sure where that comes from, or why it is the case. Maybe it's because it is something that you can't actually see… it is not a physical ailment. It has only been in the last few years that men have been starting to open up about these issues and this has been mainly due to high profile public people speaking out, which is a step in the right direction.

The hardest thing to do is to take that first step and it is also important to know that you are not showing a sign of weakness by asking for help. It actually takes great strength and courage to acknowledge that you are not coping with your current situation. When you can finally admit that you have a problem, it is like an enormous weight has been lifted off your shoulders. You are not alone and, as the saying goes, a problem shared is a problem halved.

It is easy for people to say cheer up or get over it, but for people that are suffering from depression, nothing that you can say or do makes a difference when you are in the depths of despair. The feeling of helplessness and worthlessness overpowers everything, making it difficult to see the positive side of anything in life.

It is very important for the friends and family around people affected by depression that they look out for the signs, as it is critical to the diagnosis and treatment. In most cases it is undetected or misdiagnosed. However, the sooner you can get treatment, the greater the chance of a faster recovery. The most important thing is to recognise the depression and to seek help from a professional.

Even after all of this time and the healing process, there are still moments when the depression can resurface, so it is important to feel the emotion, acknowledge it and manage it in the best way possible. This was evident recently when, out of the blue, I was contacted by a work colleague who advised me that a friend had taken his life. It later came out that he was battling the illness for close to 20 years and was suffering in silence. Now to look at him you wouldn't have picked it, so it is not always obvious. I can only imagine what he must have been going through.

It is vital to your health and wellbeing that you talk about how you're feeling with those close to you at first and then seek professional help if you're finding it difficult to cope and function day to day. Society says that men are the providers and the protectors and that they should be able to sort out their issues with a few mates over a beer, but statistics shows that this is not the case, with men taking their own lives in ridiculous numbers. We don't hear about this in the media because the subject is taboo and easy to sweep under the carpet.

If you suspect that someone you know is suffering from depression, it may be hard to know exactly what to say or do. You can start by simply talking to the person and asking them how they're feeling. Listen to what they're saying without offering any advice or suggestions. Sit in a relaxed position and maintain eye contact with them. Spending time with the person and showing them that you care can go a long way. Try and get them to open up if possible, by asking open-ended questions (something that requires more than a 'yes' or 'no' response). If the person you're talking to gets angry, it is important to stay calm and not get caught up in the emotion. Let them know that you are not judging them, but merely wanting to help them.

If they feel comfortable talking to you, assist them to make an appointment and offer to go with them to see a GP or mental health professional. If this is pushing the friendship too far, then offer to seek information for them which they can read or call a help line to discuss further, anonymously. Encourage them to exercise, eat well and get involved in social activities again. Maintain regular contact with them and encourage those close to them to do the same.

It is important not to pressure these people to 'snap out of it' or to 'get their act together' because this can have a negative effect. Do your best not to stay away from them or avoid them as they can feel unloved or unwanted, possibly even that the world will be better off without them. It is human instinct to give advice or offer suggestions, such as staying busy or to get out more, but this can be unhelpful. You can't mask the problem with drugs or alcohol and assume that the problem will just go away, so do your best to let them know that you are there to help them and be a shoulder to lean on. Sometimes you need to be firm to be kind, but tread lightly.

Even though you may be living in a bubble during the whole period from diagnosis and through treatment in a traumatic event such as we experienced, it is vitally important that you all take some time out for yourself to clear your mind and recharge your batteries, because the stress and anxiety can take its toll on you physically, mentally and emotionally, potentially leading to depression and other illnesses.

There is a hormonal response in the body when it is placed into a constant state of stress and anxiety. When there is chronic stress, the adrenalin levels remain high, which can lead to anxiety due to the constant dump of cortisol. This is turn can lead to insomnia as there is an absence of melatonin and then ultimately lead to depression because of the lack of serotonin (happy hormone).

Everyone will be different with their road to recovery, but this is what I found helped me:

- Writing a book has been therapeutic. You don't have to go to this extreme, but you may want to start a journal or diary

- Maintaining a work–life balance (speak to your employer)
- Going for a walk or a bike ride, exercising/movement/activity
- Catching up with family and friends. Get back into socialising
- Having interests or hobbies, other than with your partner/children
- Joining groups or clubs
- Talking about it, don't bottle it up inside
- Challenge DUC Club (Dad's Ultimate Challenge)
- Camp Quality family camps
- Starlight Escapes (through Starlight Children's Foundation)
- Travel, break out of the everyday routines
- Day trips with the family
- Reading positive books and listening to self-help audiobooks
- Attending workshops and seminars
- Hanging around positive people

Other things that can be useful in helping reduce stress and anxiety are avoiding major life changes during this period (i.e. moving house or changing jobs), and avoiding personal conflict. Get back to doing the things you enjoy, control your work environment and ensure you have enough time to rest and relax, having a good night's sleep, meditating or controlled breathing, muscle tension or relaxation exercises or some form of movement and staying active can relieve tension and relax your mind. Seeking help by talking to a friend, doctor, counsellor or someone else you trust can also put your mind at ease.

There is a lot of help available for depression and mental health issues, with no one treatment being right or wrong. This may involve medical intervention, psychological intervention or complimentary and lifestyle intervention. Each person will respond differently to one or more modalities and can be quick or take some time, so you will need to have patience and persistence.

You don't have to battle through your struggles on your own. It is important to have a support network around you, and more importantly know where to find them. I have included some contact details below for your reference, so please get in touch with them if you feel the need to discuss your personal issues.

Beyond Blue

1300 224 636

www.beyondblue.org.au

Black Dog Institute

(02) 9382 2991

www.blackdoginstitute.org.au

Lifeline

13 11 14

www.lifeline.org.au

MensLine Australia

1300 789 978

www.mensline.org.au

Kids Helpline

1800 551 800

www.kidshelpline.com.au

CHAPTER 5

KEEPING IT TOGETHER

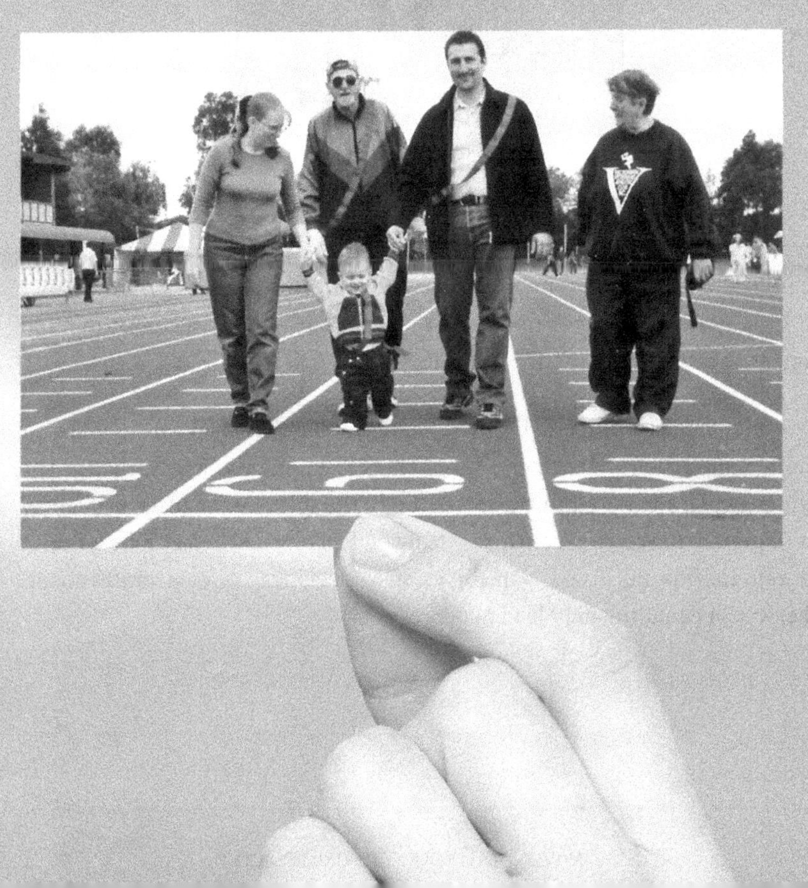

Chapter 5

Keeping It Together

(Jim)

Family is not an important thing.
It's everything

Michael J. Fox

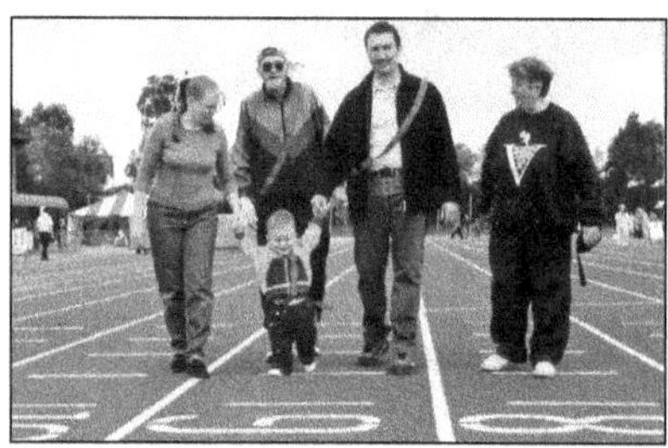

During the most difficult times of our life, it is better to go through the experience with someone by your side and I will be forever grateful that I had Lisa by mine. She was the 'rock' that kept our family together, from the moment Sam was diagnosed.

I took a lot longer to come to terms with the fact that Sam had cancer and also a significant vision impairment. Lisa was able to express and verbalise her feelings, while I suffered in silence. Nobody should have to suffer in silence. It is important to speak to someone when you feel ready, whether it be a friend you can confide in, a family member, a work colleague or a professional. Otherwise it can ultimately lead to depression.

As a couple you process things differently, so it is important to give each other space, but also to be there for one another when needed. If your spouse or partner wants to talk openly with you, don't shut them out as this can lead to a breakdown in communication with your lives going in two very different directions. Even if you don't feel like talking at the time, at least lend them an ear and just listen. It can help you see things from their perspective and assist you with the healing process.

This whole life changing experience has not only brought us closer together, but made us a lot stronger as individuals and allowed us to look at life very differently. We now appreciate the little things and 'don't sweat the small stuff'.

However, our relationship could have gone down a very different path. We spent a lot of time at the hospital waiting room and got to meet a lot of families and couples. Like us, most came together, but there were also quite a few that didn't survive the stress and turmoil of relentless visits, treatments and admissions. It can take its toll on you if you let it and don't look after yourself individually and as a couple.

Not only are there the emotional stresses, but the physical stresses can also affect your mood and ability to look for the positives, especially when you're at your lowest point. Therefore, it is extremely important for you to try and get a good night's sleep, have some time out, stay in touch with your friends and family and TRY to keep life as normal as possible. This is the key to staying balanced and being able to cope.

When you are spending so much time at hospital and in medical appointments it is difficult for both adults to go to work. This in turn can place financial pressures on the relationship and is one of the leading causes for divorce and break ups. For a period of two and a half years after Sam lost his sight, I worked two jobs (day and night) to allow Lisa the time to do what she had to and give him the time to adjust to life without vision. At that time Mitchell was only twelve months old and Lisa had just returned to work part-time from maternity leave.

In times of hardship due to medical reasons, there are organisations out there that can help you with your finances. It is just a case of knowing where to look and who to speak to. Don't be too proud to put your hand up for some assistance in your time of need. There will be a time when you can pay it forward once you have come out the other end.

It can also be difficult to remain focused and motivated to go to work when your child is constantly in and out of hospital. Speak to your employer, be open and honest and let them know what is going on, because you'll be surprised how supportive and flexible they can be. There is nothing worse than being at work and your mind is constantly wandering to your child and what they are going through.

You need to make time for each other to still be a couple. Date nights, concerts, dinners and weekends away are a good start. What brought you together in the first place? Continue doing what made you both happy and brought you joy before the illness. We had amazing support from family and friends and they understood the importance of having one on one time away from the sterile walls of the hospital.

As important as it is to spend time together, it is equally important to spend time apart, doing your own thing. Whether it be going out with a friend, joining a club of some sort, pampering yourself, or reading a book, you should make it a priority to have some down time and recharge your batteries. This will help you deal with the day to day grind and be at your best when your family needs you the most. Understand that your partner needs to do this too. Make sure that you are both getting the time you need to recharge.

Do you put the needs of everyone else before yours? Are you exhausted and totally spent of energy at the end of each day? That really has to change from today and you need to put yourself first. It is not selfish and will benefit your partner and family more than you can imagine. To keep yourself in optimum shape, have a massage, soak in a bath with essential oils, meditate, do a yoga class, go to the gym, take up a sport, catch up with friends, find a hobby, go on a retreat and have that weekend getaway you've been putting off.

One word that has defined our relationship from the very beginning is compromise. Lisa and I have come from totally different backgrounds and cultures that are poles apart, but quickly worked out that for our relationship to survive and thrive we had to learn to meet each other in the middle. It is all about mutual respect and trust where you can work through your differences and treat each other as equals. No one is right or wrong, but your point of view should be heard and respected. Sometimes you just have to agree to disagree and move on! Don't hold a grudge against your partner or spouse as this can fester into something more down the track.

Don't be afraid to show your affection to your other half or to tell them how much you love them. Send them a special message during the day, give them a hug and kiss, bring them a bunch of flowers or surprise them with a romantic dinner. If they do something out of the ordinary for you, tell them that you appreciate them and that you are extremely grateful. It doesn't take much, but it sure does go a long way. And one word of advice – don't take each other for granted.

It takes hard work and commitment to maintain a long and healthy relationship. It doesn't 'just happen'! A traumatic event can be the straw that breaks the camel's back in a marriage that already has cracks appearing. It is important to have a strong foundation and to keep growing as an individual as well as a couple. At first it may be a physical attraction or a common interest, but this is not enough to keep you together for the long term.

There is a common saying that 'life is a rollercoaster' and it couldn't be more true. Nobody gets through life unscathed and the ups and downs can come when you least expect them. Being able to meet a challenge as a couple can help the relationship become stronger and more resilient. You ask any couple that has stood the test of time.

When children come into a family, this can change the dynamic of the relationship and the household. Where your partner used to give you their undivided attention, it is now redirected towards another individual, and when you have more than one child it is split even more. Throwing a child with an illness into the equation can escalate this to the point of living separate lives, like ships passing in the night. The mother or father feels a deep sense of obligation to be there for their sick child 24/7 and forgets to make time for their partner. Make a conscious effort to set aside time for you as a couple, and when you are together give them your full attention.

Nobody is perfect, so don't expect your partner to be. Everybody has an annoying habit that gets on their partner's nerves, but don't keep going on about it. Sometimes it is better to just bite your tongue! I'm sure that you have a bad habit or two in your closet. Accept the other person for who they are and don't try to change them. They need to make a conscious decision to change themselves and more importantly, want to change.

The secret to finding true happiness in life starts with the individual. Your partner or your family are not responsible for your happiness. If you are looking to others for your happiness and don't get it, then this can lead to resentment, disappointment and a lack of fulfilment. If you can't be happy within yourself, then how can you be happy around others? Think about what you are grateful for and count your blessings, because each day above ground is a good day… if you truly believe it.

What is your story and do you allow that to define you? Are you the mum with the sick kid, the guy who lost his leg in an accident, the woman who beat breast cancer?

All of our stories have a beginning, middle, and end. Are you living in the past, the present or the future? Do you keep reliving your trauma over and over and find it hard to move on? Are you constantly thinking about what is going to happen in the future? If you feel that you are stuck within your thoughts, and keep going over and over them in your head, why not live in the now and be mindful of the present. It is the best way to live life to the fullest and truly experience all that life has to offer. Take a few deep breaths and give it a try.

From my experience, it is best to show your emotions and let them all out, because holding them inside is unhealthy for you and those around you. As hard as it may seem at the time, share how you're feeling. You will feel a tremendous weight lift off your shoulders.

It could be in the way of keeping a journal if you feel uncomfortable verbalising it to anyone else, or alternatively speak to a friend, a family member, a health professional, a counsellor, a psychologist or even a support group. There are lots of people out there who are willing to help.

If you are feeling sad, cry. If you are feeling happy, laugh. If you are feeling angry, shout. We both experienced grief, which included a wide range of emotions, thoughts and behaviours. At the end of the day we are human beings with feelings and emotions and should be exactly that and not cold, lifeless robots.

Another important factor that helped us remain sane was our involvement with the wonderful charities such as Starlight Children's Foundation, Camp Quality, Challenge and Ronald McDonald House Charities. Not only were they a fantastic resource for the children, but they were also a vital support network for the adults. We were able to meet other families going through a similar experience and could understand exactly how they felt. We could share our stories and watch the kids smiling, laughing and having fun at the same time. Without even knowing it, this was a form of therapy. I'm just sorry that we didn't make contact with them sooner, because we didn't start using their services until near the very end of Sam's treatment.

If you are struggling to be on the same page as your partner, then you may need to seek some professional help such as counselling. This does not mean the end, and to the contrary can save your marriage. Sometimes it is difficult to express exactly how you feel and you only need some guidance to draw it out of you. The art of knowing when to ask for help will be your saviour.

CHAPTER 6

HOSPITAL

THE PEOPLE WHO WORK THERE AND HOW TO SURVIVE IT

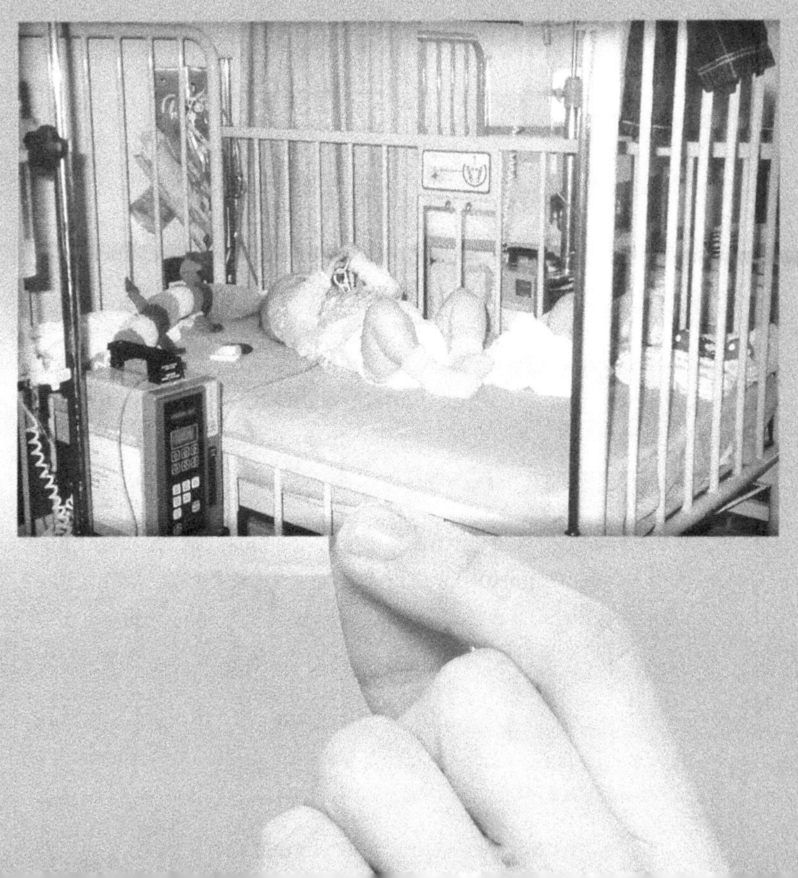

Chapter 6

Hospital – The People Who Work There And How to Survive It

(Lisa)

> *Listen to your body. It gives you warning signs when something is not right.*
>
> **Jim Valavanis**

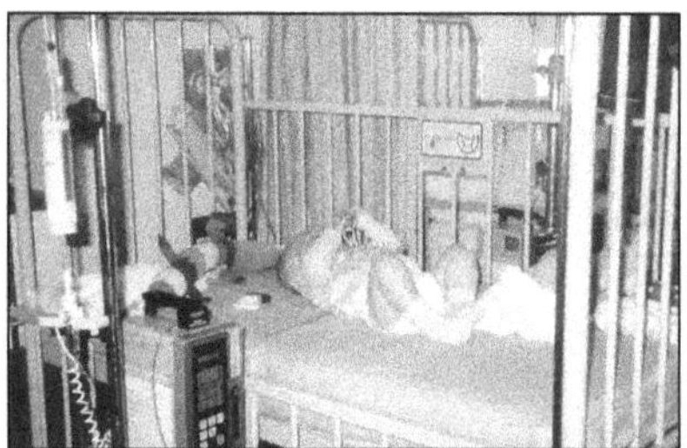

While writing this book, one of our aims is, hopefully, to clear a bit of the fog related to subjects that we have talked about, such as retinoblastoma, grief and hospital. We have thought about information that may have helped us along the way when we were going through it all. In saying this, to follow are a few points that we thought may be helpful relating to hospital and the medical interventions we experienced in general.

Hospital. This can be a very scary word, not only for kids, but for adults also. It's scary enough when we go to hospital for ourselves, but if we are there because of our own children, it can be an absolutely terrifying experience.

Jim and I were relatively healthy people. Apart from the occasional day surgery for very minor issues, or for me going to hospital to give birth to Sam, we had never really had any need to go to hospitals for any length of time. Suddenly, when Sam was diagnosed, we were thrown into a whole new life of endless hospital appointments and admissions. And the madness of busy hospital visits would continue for the first nearly five years of Sam's life. Even though now the hospital regime has calmed down, Sam will still need to have regular appointments and tests, possibly for a very long time. Just recently Sam had a day at hospital consisting of an ultrasound, MRI and x-ray. The fun never ends.

Sam's very first hospital appointment at the Royal Children's Hospital in Melbourne was on the day that he was diagnosed. His first admission involved a general anaesthetic, CT scan, ultrasound and lumbar puncture. All of this at the grand old age of three months. That was the worst day of Jim's and my life.

However, this was just the start of things to come. Between that first admission and when he turned five years old, Sam had more than 100 general anaesthetics, admissions to three different hospitals, numerous tests in different departments, endless 'take home' medications and eye drops, minor and major surgeries, both day admissions and admissions of up to a week in length, internal prosthesis implanted, removal of infected internal prosthesis, chemotherapy, radiation therapy, cryotherapy, laser treatment, CT scans, ultrasounds, injections directly into his eye, moulds taken for prosthetic eyes and two enucleations.

For years before Sam's diagnosis, Jim and I had always donated to the Royal Children's Hospital Good Friday Appeal, thinking what an amazing hospital it was to help so many sick children and support their families. Little did we realise that we would soon become 'Frequent Flyers' there.

Every fourth Wednesday we nicknamed 'Eye Day'. That was when there would be a theatre list for kids either with Rb or kids with a parent with the disease or the Rb gene. The day would start by waking Sam up and feeding him as soon as possible before the cut off time, when pre-anaesthetic fasting would begin. We would go in to the Royal Children's Hospital and check in to the Day Surgery department. Then the waiting would begin. The kids would be put under anaesthetic and be taken into theatre one at a time. There was anywhere up to 16 kids on 'the list'. I would always ask when we got there where Sam was on the list. The doctors would tend to put the younger babies and kids, and also newly diagnosed cases at the start of the list. When I would ask the nurses in Day Surgery where Sam was placed, it was usually last or second last on the list. That meant a long wait.

The waiting was always very hard and extremely draining, especially for us as parents. Sam and the other kids would never stay still while waiting. Thankfully, there was usually a stash of toys to entertain the kids. Mind you, sharing with all of the other kids the amount of toys that were there was a bit tricky, especially when most of the toys or puzzles were either broken or missing parts. Quite often in Day Surgery they would have a Music Therapist or Play Therapist visit while making their way around the hospital. This would be a good distraction from the long wait, all be it a short distraction. Sometimes also, if we knew that we were near the end of the theatre list, we would be able to walk around the hospital, or even visit 'The Starlight Room', with the nurses sending us off with a pager, to let us know when they needed us back at Day Surgery.

But it was always still a long day, especially when you have a tired and hungry child, who doesn't really understand why they aren't allowed to eat anything. We would always wait until Sam went in to theatre before we would go off to eat, so we would share his hunger. It wasn't unheard of to have to fast Sam from 7 am, be admitted to Day Surgery at 12 pm, then to have him not go in to theatre until 5 pm. He would then be in theatre for 30–45 minutes, while the doctors would check any changes to the tumours in his eyes and administer treatment if it was required. We would get worried if he would be in there a little longer than usual. This quite often either meant that the doctors had found something new, or that they had to do treatment. They would then bring Sam out to recovery and get us to come in once he was stabilised. More often than not, Sam would come out of the anaesthetic angry, especially if he woke up to find a cannula still in his hand.

Sam would need to have something to eat and drink before we were allowed to leave for home. However, if Sam had received cryotherapy treatment in theatre, he would be in a huge amount of pain and just not want to have anything. There was also a balancing act with the anaesthetic, getting the right balance of anti-nausea and pain relief drugs while under anaesthetic, otherwise getting home could take longer if he was sick in the recovery room. I clearly remember one rainy dark night driving home with him when he was quite young, having to pull over on the side of the road around Albert Park Lake to clean up the 'mess' of the anaesthetic aftermath that he had totally covered himself with on the way home. I would quite often call Jim from the hospital before we would leave for home, telling him to "Get the towels ready". This meant that Jim would cover Sam's bed in towels, as he would spend a lot of the night vomiting. It was never usually a fun night after a huge day at the hospital.

I used to say to Jim that it was so tiring just sitting around and doing nothing. And we would do that trip with Sam once every four weeks. This went on for over four years.

The Royal Children's Hospital in Melbourne is an amazing place. The day Sam was diagnosed, we walked in there thinking we knew who we were, and walked out some hours later completely different people. We have spent lots of hours in that hospital, in waiting rooms trying to entertain a tired, hungry and frustrated child while waiting for treatment or surgery. We have shed bucket loads of tears there, some happy but most sad. We have felt sorry for Sam and ourselves there, but also seen many other children with their families that have made us realise that we are so lucky and incredibly grateful for the hand that life has dealt our family, knowing that the situation could have been much worse.

While at the 'RCH' we have spoken to lots of other families, whether other Rb families or parents of children there for other reasons. In a strange way, I looked forward to hospital days as a chance to catch up with other families with whom we had shared a journey. Many we had met while Sam was quite young and newly diagnosed. It was good to be able to talk to other families who had travelled the road that we had just started on. Although every diagnosis and treatment plan is not exactly the same, it was nice to talk to people that had 'been there'.

We went in to hospital with Sam once a month and be greeted by many staff members who became like a weird second family to Sam. It was always good to see familiar faces, made it feel a little less daunting. The staff there saw Sam from a three month old newly diagnosed baby to a four-and-a-half-year-old boy, and beyond. And for us as parents this was comforting. Although we did see a lot of different nurses in the hospital, many of the ones we saw in Day Surgery were the same ones that were there from month to month. They saw Sam grow up, but also got to know us, which made it easy to talk to them about how both Sam and we were doing. The consistency and familiarity of faces was reassuring for all of us. Just recently Sam had an appointment with the 'Long Term Follow Up Clinic', a once a year appointment with an oncologist, endocrinologist, psychologist and dietician. The nurse who was in with the oncologist was a nurse whom we hadn't seen for years, as she administered Sam's chemo to him when he was three months old, 13 years ago. It felt like meeting up with an old friend!

I have a great admiration for the people who work at the RCH. I don't think that we have encountered anybody who works there who was not friendly or supportive or made us feel at ease. It's a special kind of person that works there.

The specialised doctors who have treated Sam along the way, well, I cannot even put into words what they have meant to us. Both the Oncologists and the Ophthalmology Doctors and Orthoptist/Care Coordinator that we have had treat Sam have been wonderful. These were the specific medical specialists who treated Sam on a regular basis.

When Sam was first diagnosed, we were thrown straight into an unfamiliar world, full of confusion and uncertainty. We had been abruptly given a diagnosis, which then implanted the idea that it was all over for Sam or any chance of sight for him from that day onwards. But once we were able to sit down with the doctors and Rb coordinator, they were able to give us some sense of hope. All along throughout this journey, I feel as though it has been a team effort to save our son. We needed to work as a team with all of the health professionals involved. We were all trying to fight the same battle together. They were able to help and support us and Sam in many ways, some of which, not all medical staff can successfully do.

Along our way through the cancer journey, I did learn a lot about many functions of the hospitals that Sam visited and the staff that treated him. From the doctors to the nurses, the anaesthetists to the ward staff, we learnt so much along the way. We learnt about the routines of the wards, the different treatment processes, hospital 'slang' or terminology, the personality differences of the doctors and the reasoning behind tests, diagnosis and the decisions on treatment regimes.

After talking with other families who have been with us along this long road, or families in similar circumstances, I wanted to cover situations that can make it a much harder, already difficult experience.

Speak Up

I think that one of our aims of this book is to tell people to trust their gut instincts. If something doesn't feel right, question it. One of the most important and invaluable thing that I learnt through this entire process is that doctors and medical professionals do not know everything and are not always correct. I learnt that as parents we could and should question the health professionals if we are unsure or not satisfied with their opinion, diagnosis or treatment plan.

I have also realised that I am allowed to speak up if I am not happy with what I have been told. To the doctor, your child may just be a 20-minute appointment in the middle of a busy day. To a parent, it is your child, your life, your world. Get a second, third or fourth opinion. At the end of the day, if you are wrong and there is not a problem, then what does it matter? But if you don't follow it up and there is something wrong…

At our post birth paediatrician appointment for Sam, the doctor didn't think there was anything wrong with Sam's vision. "It can take babies up to twelve weeks to focus" were his exact words. It was only through showing our concerns and questioning our local Health Centre Nurse, that she paid attention to us and got us in to an appointment with a paediatric ophthalmologist. If we hadn't looked further into it and simply trusted this 'professional', Sam would most probably have died.

Something that I really liked through Sam's treatment was that, although we worked primarily with one Ophthalmologist, he worked hand in hand with another Ophthalmologist. There were quite a few situations along the way when we just weren't sure about the decision that needed to be made regarding treatment. If we wanted him to, the other Ophthalmologist would sit down with us and give us his opinion on what he thought was an appropriate plan of attack, even if it was different to Sam's Ophthalmologist's opinion.

During Sam's EUAs at the Royal Children's Hospital, there were quite a few months in a row that I would have a heated discussion with the same anaesthetist who would put him under. He would say that the best way to put Sam under anaesthetic would be by the needle. I disagreed with him, knowing that Sam used to totally freak out when anybody would come near him with a needle. I found that the best way he coped being put off to sleep was by the gas mask, or as he called it, the 'chocolate mask'. He called it this because the anaesthetic assistant or nurse would put a chocolate-smelling essence in the mask so it would smell nicer for the kids than the gas coming through it. It was one time that I was in with Sam to have his anaesthetic, that the anaesthetist tried the needle approach. After a lot of screaming from Sam and blood spurting everywhere after a failed attempt at inserting the needle, I knew it was time for me to assert my 'Mummy-ness'. From that point onwards, Sam was put under anaesthetic with the 'chocolate mask'.

If tests are required, or a course of treatment, understand what is involved and what it is for. Be aware of any possible side effects, risks, or long term effects. With Sam's chemotherapy and radiation therapy, we had to weigh up the benefits of having the treatment, given that two possible long term effects of both of these treatments was an increased risk of secondary cancer and/or possible hearing loss.

Medical Jargon

Holy crap! How I wish I had done that medical degree before I had kids. Jim and I have learned so much about the eye, cancer and cancer treatments. But at the start of it all, when the doctors explained things to us, they may as well have been speaking Martian! I realised very quickly that if I wanted to understand what was happening to Sam, then I had to ask the doctors to stop using 'big words'. I didn't care if the doctors thought I was dumb, I needed to understand what was going on in words that I could understand. I learnt not to be afraid to ask questions. Do not end an appointment or meeting without being fully aware of what is going on. Which leads to…

Stupid Questions

I am the queen of stupid questions. But I think I agree with the statement, please excuse my paraphrasing, that the only stupid question is the one that you don't ask. I have gotten to the point in my life that I don't care what people think about me. What matters is what I think of me. And if I am unsure about something, I will ask, no matter how stupid the question sounds. I remember Sam's oncologist reiterating that to us. I know I feel more stupid if I don't ask when I am unsure about something, and walk away being none the wiser.

The doctors at hospital made us feel comfortable enough to be able to ask whatever we needed to, to totally be happy that we understood what was happening or what needed to be done.

Questions in General

The whole concept of hospital can be a little terrifying. So lots of questions might arise. We were so quickly thrown into the cancer spiral after Sam was diagnosed, that we hardly had time to think. A lot of other parents have also found that, finding there seems to be no time to even stop and breathe. So, below are a few questions that might come up for you, that you may not think of at the time. They are in no particular order, just happens to be the way they poured out for me while writing.

- Ask what tests and procedures are for, if you don't know or understand
- Ask what is involved with the test or procedure.
- Are there side effects or risks involved with what is being done.
- If you are unsure if a symptom, reaction to treatment, or anything is 'normal', ask.
- How long will treatment be for?
- Is there support or somebody that you can speak to, i.e. Social Worker or Pastoral support.
- If you are wanting to incorporate natural therapies or alternative therapies, speak to the medical specialists about that.
- Where can you find more information about the condition, procedure or treatment.
- Are there alternative options to the treatment or procedure being suggested?
- What is the difference between going into hospital as a private or a public patient?

- Are you able to get a second opinion?
- Can you speak with other people or families with the same condition?
- Who will be performing the procedure or treatment?
- Is there an anaesthetic involved?
- Can you go in to have your child put under anaesthetic?
- How long will recovery take?
- Who can be contacted after discharge from hospital if there are any concerns, questions or problems?
- What should you bring with you for a hospital stay?

Other Little Bits of Advice

If I can impart any words of wisdom from our experiences, or just simply ideas that may help, then hopefully I may make the fog over hospital stays seem a little clearer. Here are some of my ideas.

- If it is your child in hospital, stay with them if possible. I have always stayed with Sam while he has needed to stay in hospital, or if I couldn't, Jim did. Not only am I there for him, but I know that it is reassuring for myself that I am there for when any tests are to be taken, e.g., blood tests or x-rays, or for when the doctors come around.
- Be aware but not alarmed. I know in our case, this related to Jim 'Googling' retinoblastoma. When Sam was first diagnosed, Jim decided to look into the cancer on Google. I went downstairs to our study to find him crying over the computer. That was the worst thing he could do, as he was of course looking into the worst case scenarios. Ask the people who are handling your individual situation.

- Disclose as much information as you have available to you. Do not leave any details out, no matter how small or irrelevant you think they are. Let all the health professionals in your 'team' know about each other and other treatments that are happening simultaneously and in the past. Let them be aware of all medications, alternative treatments or therapies, vitamins, etc.

- If there are other people or families who have children that have been through the same diagnosis/treatment, speak with them.

- Ask as many questions as you need to.

However, in saying all that I have about hospital, it is one of Sam's favourite places to visit. Sam thought of hospital as his 'Luna Park' and still thinks of it as a magical place. I think it is because he has grown up knowing nothing else, not realising that this is not the way that life should be. He has always felt safe and comfortable about going to the RCH, and I know that it is because of the people that have been a part of our story there. And for that I say thank you.

CHAPTER 7

THOSE WHO HELPED SAM SEE

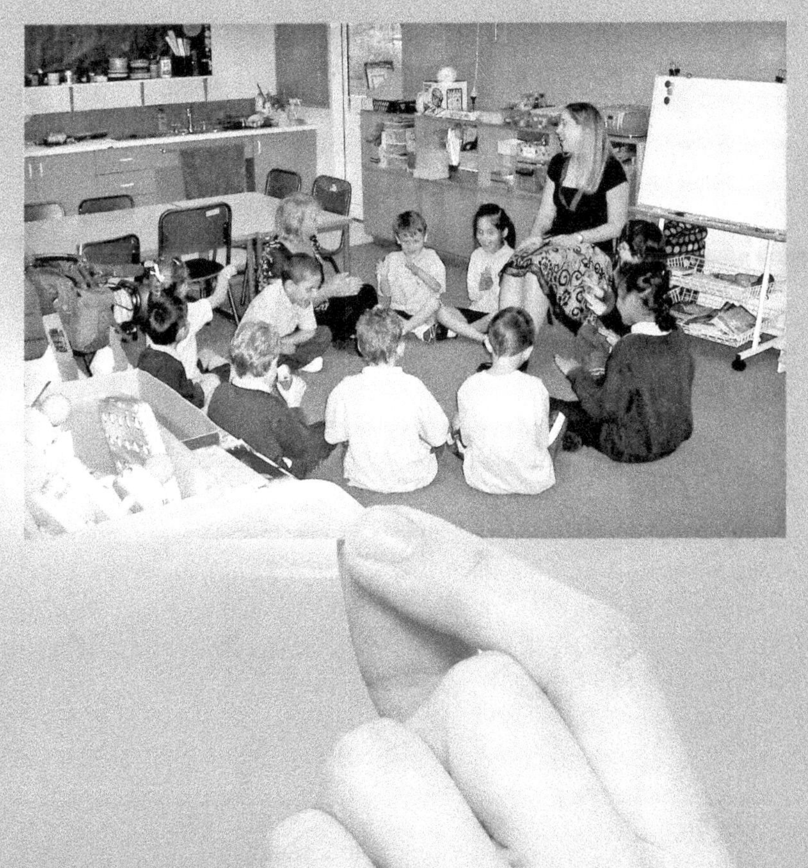

Chapter 7

Those Who Helped Sam See

(Lisa)

> *Don't let what you cannot do interfere with what you can do.*
>
> **John Wooden – NCAA Basketball Coach**

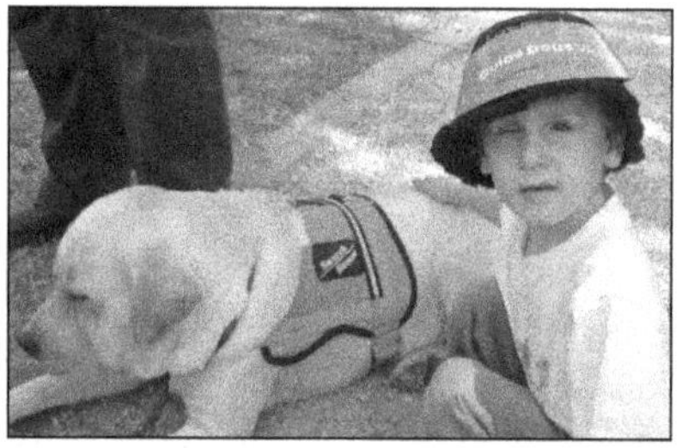

"My baby's going to be blind", then I burst into tears. That is how I introduced myself to RVIB (Royal Victorian Institute for the Blind, now Vision Australia). The day after Sam was diagnosed, I went straight into panic and fix-it mode. I had heard of RVIB in the past, always watched the RVIB Carols by Candlelight every Christmas Eve. I knew that they helped blind people, but other than that, I didn't know any more. I just knew that we needed help.

That day, I looked at the phone book and found RVIB in there. I contacted one of the suburban offices that was located near where we lived at the time. The wonderful Sandy answered the phone and copped the full force of my tears. But looking back now, that was the best thing that I could have ever done. It felt like from that day on RVIB stepped in to save the day. No sooner did I bare my soul, than it felt like things were going to be okay.

Our first face to face contact with RVIB was an Early Childhood Educator named Judy. Judy met Sam and I when we were still newly diagnosed, during the time when my head was still spinning. Judy would come out to visit us at home once a fortnight. We would greet her at the front door, with her basket of goodies for Sam to explore. Judy was there to help Sam until he ventured off to start school. She would play with him, playing with puzzles, feeling shapes, lying in the 'little room' to help him develop his sense of spatial awareness, and to teach him to use the limited amount of vision he did have. She would work with him to get him sitting, crawling and walking. Judy was there to help him grow and develop to the best of his ability, despite his vision impairment. She was his first contact to the world of braille, introducing him to a Perkins Brailler. She also introduced him to the Feelix Library, the 'feely' books were the start of his love of stories.

When it came time to head off to kinder, Judy was still there for him. Along with the amazing kinder staff at Patterson Lakes Kindergarten, she worked with Sam to make the transition into an educational environment as easy as possible. She would come out to visit Sam at kinder, alternating with home visits, to make a challenging kinder year a memorable one for him. Sam lost his second eye during his kinder year, so having Judy there for not only Sam, but also the other children and the staff, was invaluable.

But I think what I remember most about this time we had with Judy is how she was there for me. Judy and I would discuss how Sam's treatment was going. I would discuss my thoughts and fears with her, how I was feeling about what was going on. There was one night that she came out to our home. It was just before Sam's final eye surgery to remove his second eye. We had our parents there for Judy to speak with us all. She talked to us about what would happen, how to support and help Sam, and how to support each other. That was an incredibly hard situation that was made slightly better for the fact that Judy was there.

For me, Judy was there as my saviour. She would help me to work with Sam, give me ideas for toys for him, an ear to listen to me, a shoulder to cry on when things got too much, and a wealth of support and information to help guide me through the disability minefield. But most of all, she was a friend. I know that during those first five years of Sam's life would have been very different if it were not for Judy. How do you thank somebody for that?

After kinder, it was time to jump into the big wide world of school. As a parent, this is a scary time, when your baby goes off to start the next phase of their life. But even more so when life can be so uncertain with a disability thrown into the equation. It was not just a case of throwing him in to the local Government Primary School, like you may do with a regular child. Judy had suggested the Vision Australia School in Burwood. Immediately I got my back up. My first thought was that I didn't want him going there. In my mind, by sending him there I was admitting to myself that my child was disabled. Well DDAAHHHHH!!!!!! Even though I knew it, it was still hard to say it and admit it to myself. I initially thought that he could go to mainstream school and the VA school, both part-time. But after sitting down and thinking about it sensibly, we realised that he needed to be at the VA school full time. And now, looking back, we could not have made a better decision. Sam was there for Prep full time, and Grade One, integrating between there and mainstream school. The school closed down at the end of Sam's Grade One year. As he had just become totally blind the year before starting there, it was the best thing to have him there, full time. He was fully immersed into braille, orientation and mobility, and other skills that only blind or vision impaired children need to focus on. There was Music with Sue, Art with Michael, Technology with Garry, Sport with Emily. And the wonderful work that his teachers Marg P, Marg R and Ondina provided. He also had access to other services such as physiotherapy, occupational therapy, speech therapy and daily living skills. If he was at a mainstream school during that first year at school, he would have to take time out from his everyday school time to have this support and specialised teaching. Looking back at Sam's time at the VA school, we could not have wished for a better start to an education.

Vision Australia have helped with many other essential services throughout Sam's life. We've all seen them around, the white cane that blind people use.

To Sam, this is an absolutely essential tool to help him with his independence. But how do you use the thing? He has worked with a few different Orientation and Mobility Instructors, Marg and Gail, since he started using a cane, about nine or so years ago. His cane means that Sam is able to move around familiar and new environments with confidence and independence. Sam has had many canes along the way, he has this terrible habit of growing and outgrowing them. Unfortunately, Sam has been the demise of a cane or two also. We have had Sam bring his cane home from school, on a bit of a different angle to how it originally went to school. I would ask him what had happened to it. "I don't know", would come the response. After discussion with teachers at school, we discovered that Sam would take out his frustrations about the differences between him and the other school kids on his cane. It is one thing that stands out as a visible sign that he is different.

There are so many people from Vision Australia who have helped both Sam and us over the years. Some services from Vision Australia which he had in the past will continue long into the future, as his needs grow and change. There are not enough words to thank Vision Australia for what they have given and done, not only for Sam, but our family.

Statewide Vision Resource Centre

Once Sam finished at the Vision Australia School, he was then full time at mainstream school. Berwick Chase Primary School was a great school for Sam. We were so lucky with the way things worked out. This school opened the same year as Sam's Grade One, so he started there in his integration year. He was the first student enrolled at the school. He stayed there to finish Grade Six. However, Sam still needed help and support in other areas that a mainstream school could not help him with.

Since being at mainstream school, along with a Teacher's/Integration Aid, Sam has had a Visiting Teacher from Statewide Vision Resource Centre (SVRC) come to support him and his teacher/aid at school. Without this support, school would be a lot more difficult for Sam. His visiting teacher for the last five years or so, Melissa, had been invaluable. She would visit Sam twice a week at school. She helped Sam – but also his teachers. She helped prepare work in a format for him, such as braille, enabling him to do the same work the rest of his class were doing. At the end of last year, Melissa moved on to work with other students. She has been greatly missed by Sam and me. Since the start of Year 8, Sam has been with another visiting teacher, Sue. Both Melissa and Sue have been a great help for Sam, but a wealth of knowledge and information for me.

Sam has also been attending Statewide Vision Resource Centre in Donvale for a number of years. He started attending 'Dot Power' sessions in his younger primary school years. This is a program to help blind or low vision children with their braille skills, in an environment that is fun. They learn through games, activities and songs. From the SVRC website: "Dot Power is to develop skills in braille and tactual graphics. Dot Power is extremely valuable because the whole learning group is collaboratively immersed in a braille-rich environment".

Sam now attends SVRC twice a term for 'Support Skills'. He loves going to these sessions. SVRC states that "This is a specialised educational program for students with vision impairments". Support skills, firstly, provides an opportunity for students to develop peer group networks with other students with vision impairments. SVRC also offers additional recreational and educational experiences that may not be available within the regular school curriculum. The program involves subjects such as maths, art, technology, sport and music. The students also have subjects like daily living skills, where they may do simple things, such as learn to make a sandwich and cut it in half, something that other kids their age may not even need to think twice about doing. An orientation and mobility instructor from Guide Dogs Victoria also goes out to SVRC to help the kids with their cane and mobility skills. Sam has also been on a number of excursions with SVRC, including going in to the Melbourne Recital Centre, where the students listened to music and were able to feel the different instruments. Sam loves his support skills sessions at SVRC, and most importantly, they have fun.

SVRC are also working quietly in the background when it comes to Sam's education. Out at Donvale, the SVRC staff produce all of the textbooks for school children in a Braille format. Even when it comes to geography, they produce tactile maps for students to feel. They will be there to support Sam until he finishes his education, through high school and even into university. Let's hope he still needs their services then, on his way to becoming a doctor or lawyer.

Guide Dogs Victoria

Oh, how I love a visit out to Guide Dogs Victoria in Kew. I cannot leave their complex without wanting to take home a few cuddly puppies. But it's not about me. Guide Dogs offer children's mobility services to blind or low vision kids. I found the following on the Guide Dogs Victoria website, which I thought summed up their program perfectly: "Orientation and Mobility is a dynamic process in which new learning builds upon established skills. As with other life skills, it is important for children to continue strengthening their orientation and mobility skills as they develop along with understanding of concepts relating to their world. This includes knowledge of body concepts and how they relate to spatial and environmental concepts. Participation in the orientation and mobility programs encourages children to develop their confidence and independent thinking skills. Children are given the opportunity to explore, problem solve and seek answers for themselves". The support that Guide Dogs provides helps to improve the children's confidence and independence in many areas of life. Sam has been lucky to be able to go to Guide Dogs at Kew for residential camps there. He has had all sorts of adventures on the camps, including going on excursions into the city and riding different forms of public transport, learning to use these safely and independently. While the kids are staying out at the residential facility at Kew, they also help with daily living activities, such as preparing food. The skills that Guide Dogs Victoria help to develop within the kids are something that can never be taught in a classroom, but are vital to help these children survive in the big wide world. Thank you Guide Dogs Victoria.

CHAPTER 8

BEYOND SIGHT FAMILY FUN DAYS

Come and Join Sam for a day full of Music, Entertainment & Fun at the...
BEYOND SIGHT
Family Fun Day
Saturday 21st April
10am – 4pm 2007
Patterson Lakes Primary School
Gladesville Boulevard, Patterson Lakes
Shrek Jumping Castle
MEGA RAFFLE • KIDS RIDES
Harley Rides (12-2pm)
ANIMAL FARM • HUGE Rock Wall
Emergency Services Displays
Food & Goodies Stalls
and much, much more...
The "Entertainment Book" for Sale
All money raised on the day will be donated to "Beyond Sight" – the auxiliary and support group for children, and therefore families suffering from Retinoblastoma Beyond Sight will put the money towards the purchase of a "RetCam" for the Royal Children's Hospital Melbourne Opthalmology Department, at a cost of $170,000.
Sam's fight for sight will soon be over.
So come along for one very important reason...
to join Sam and have some fun!
Any queries, or if you can help out in any way please contact Lisa 0412 992 618 or Rebecca 0417 500 299
BEYOND SIGHT

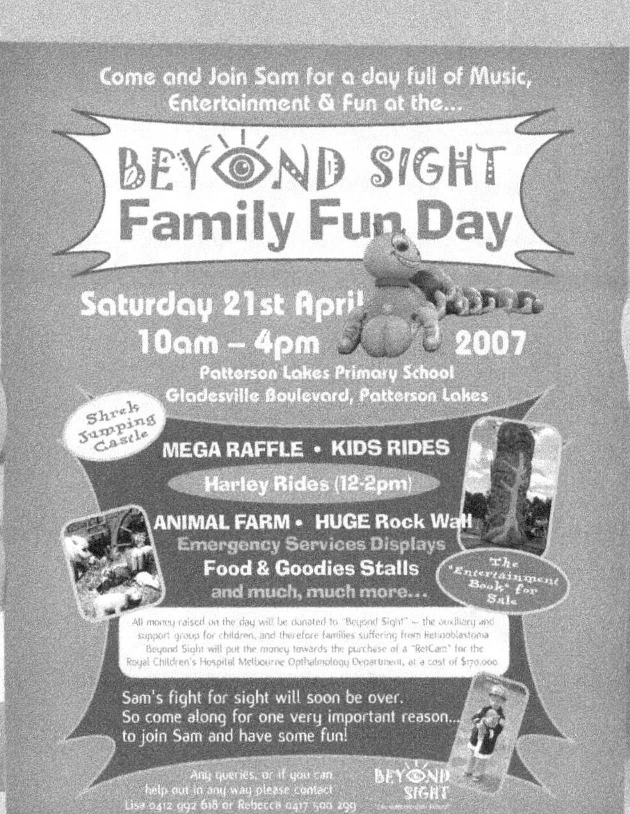

Chapter 8

Beyond Sight Family Fun Days

(Lisa)

> *It always seems impossible, until it's done.*
>
> **Nelson Mandela**

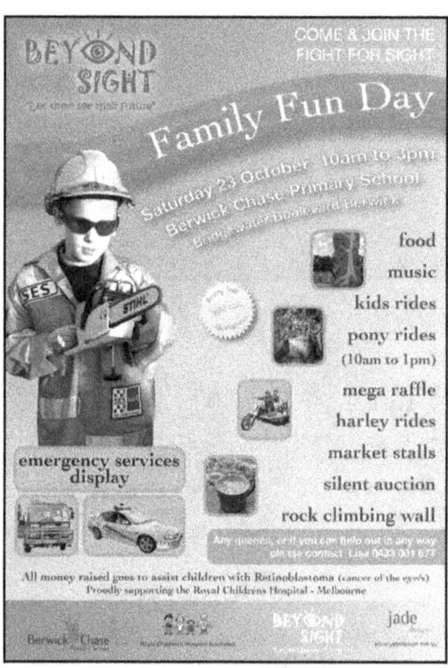

BEYOND SIGHT
COME & JOIN THE FIGHT FOR SIGHT
Family Fun Day
Saturday 23 October 10am to 3pm
Berwick Chase Primary School
food
music
kids rides
pony rides
(10am to 1pm)
mega raffle
harley rides
market stalls
silent auction
rock climbing wall
emergency services display
SES
STIHL
All money raised goes to assist children with Retinoblastoma (cancer of the eye/s)
Proudly supporting the Royal Childrens Hospital - Melbourne
Berwick Chase
jade

Beyond Sight Family Fun Days. A good idea in theory, an absolute monster of an event to organise. Let me tell you how the concept came about.

The year was 2007. Sam had already had one eye removed, and we were told that his other eye would also have to be removed, it was just a matter of when.

With this weighing heavily on my mind, I went off to bed and started to dream. I dreamt about a party to send Sam's vision off in style. In the dream, we were having a party in the street where we lived with all of our family and friends around us. When I woke up, it started…

What started as a dream soon became something very special. The dream was really burning in me and it was something that I really wanted to do for my boy. We knew that he only had limited time left to see, so I wanted to make the last visions he ever had memorable ones. My ideas that I now had from my dream grew rather quickly.

Through our meeting other families and talking to the Rb Doctors at the hospital, we were told about Beyond Sight. Beyond Sight is an auxiliary of the Royal Children's Hospital. It was created by two Rb families a number of years before Sam was diagnosed. Both families had a young son who was diagnosed with Rb around the same time. After seeing how the diagnosis and regular monitoring was done by the Doctors and the equipment that they were using, they realised that there was a need for upgraded technology and machines. And so Beyond Sight was born, an auxiliary to raise money for much needed equipment for the Ophthalmology Department. But Beyond Sight is also a support network for Rb families to be able to interact and support each other. I know that this group made a huge difference to how we first coped when going through Sam's diagnosis and treatment. When he was first diagnosed, we felt so alone and isolated, this group helped push some of those thoughts to the back of our minds. And meeting other children who had been through what Sam was now going through made us see that there could be a bright future.

What if I could make the most of 'Sam's party' and support Beyond Sight at the same time? So the concept of the 'Beyond Sight Family Fun Day' came about. So I set about creating a day to be remembered. After sharing my idea for the Family Fun Day, and the short time frame that I had to organise it in, about three months, I had some wonderful neighbours offer to lend a hand where they could. So with no background in event management, but a dream, it all started to take shape.

I liked the idea of a street party, but thought that would not work logistically. So I needed to find somewhere else to do it. We had a park area behind our house, so I thought about holding it there. I looked into this, but as it was council land, rather than private property, that wouldn't work. I approached the local primary school and told them my plan. I asked if they would consider us being able to use their outdoor grassed area for our event. They were more than happy to help out. With the tireless help from my amazing friend and neighbour Rebecca, we arranged amusement rides, food vans, an animal farm, Harley rides, Emergency Services displays, market stalls, and displays from organisations such as Vision Australia and Starlight Foundation. We had a raffle full of prizes and a silent auction, both with items graciously donated by local businesses, family and friends. We had organised media, both local newspaper and Channel 9 News. Along the way through the organising process, people and businesses were passing on donations to be put towards Beyond Sight.

So after many late nights on the computer, letters to possible donors, and feeling like the phone was permanently attached to my ear, on Saturday 21st April 2007 the first Beyond Sight Family Fun Day took place. What a day! I felt like I didn't stop throughout the entire event. The day was going really well, but then the heavens opened up and it absolutely poured down for the rest of the day. Luckily we were through most of the event when it started to rain. The raffle and silent auction were held crammed under cover.

Despite how the day ended, thanks to amazing family, friends and the local community, the day was a huge success. We were able to donate around $25,000 to Beyond Sight. But just as importantly, if not more so for me, we were able to give Sam an amazing party to remember forever. About two weeks later Sam lost his sight, but he would always have the memories of that day.

The first Beyond Sight Family Fun Day was a massive day, but the lead up and preparation of the event was incredibly exhausting. However, looking back now, I think that it helped me through an incredibly traumatic time of Sam's cancer journey. With Sam's eye removal and impending loss of sight just weeks after the event, I know that the preparation and organisation of the day kept my mind busy and gave me a sense of purpose. I can now look back and know that without doing this, I would have just been thinking of what was ahead and fallen deeper into my abyss.

So what do you do when you look back at an exhausting experience such as that? You decide to do it all again, of course! So began the creation of the second Beyond Sight Family Fun Day.

On the 23rd October 2010, it all happened again. By then we were now living in Berwick, with Sam attending Berwick Chase Primary School. With the help and support of the school's amazing Principal, Murray, we arranged to hold it on the grounds of the school. With a group of incredible school mums, especially the highly driven Adina, we went about arranging the day. Again with the great support from family, friends and local and other businesses, we put together a raffle and silent auction.

The day came around. We had amusement rides, a jumping castle, animal farm, Harley rides, food vans, market stalls, displays from Vision Australia and Guide Dogs Victoria, Emergency Services displays, merchandise from the Royal Children's Hospital for sale, and lots more. What is it with me and rain? Again, it poured, but unlike the first event, most of the market stalls, silent auction and raffle were under cover in the school hall.

So again, with the amazing help we received from family, friends and the local community, we had another successful day, raising close to $10,000 to donate to Beyond Sight.

Looking back at both of the Beyond Sight Family Fun Days, I often wonder if I would ever organise another one. My initial reaction is "Hell NO!!!". But, I should never say never. One day I may have a momentary lapse of sanity and commit myself to doing it again. The first one started as a celebration and party for Sam, but by the time the second event was over, it had come to mean a lot more. We have been so grateful to Beyond Sight for what the auxiliary had done for Sam and our family. I know without the money previously raised by Beyond Sight, which has bought equipment for the Ophthalmology department at the RCH, the way that Sam was diagnosed and monitored may have been very different. I felt so honoured to be able to give back to Beyond Sight, knowing that what we have done could help other children and families in years to come.

Looking back at both of the Beyond Sight Family Fun Days, there were so many people who helped us along the way in the organisation, preparation and execution of the events. There are way too many to thank individually, but I would like to thank you all collectively. Without everybody's help, guidance, support, experience and sanity when mine had left me, these days would not have taken place. I cannot quantify my appreciation and what you all meant to me for your support. Thank you.

CHAPTER 9

THOSE WHO HAVE HELPED US

THE CHARITIES

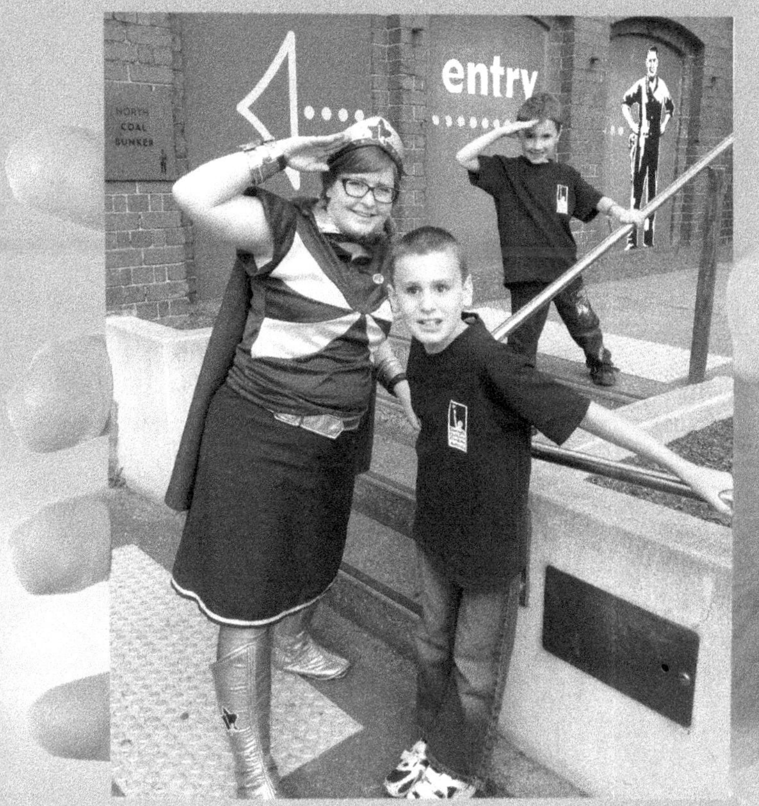

Chapter 9

Those Who Have Helped Us – The Charities

(Lisa)

Laughter is the best medicine.

Unknown
(Camp Quality slogan)

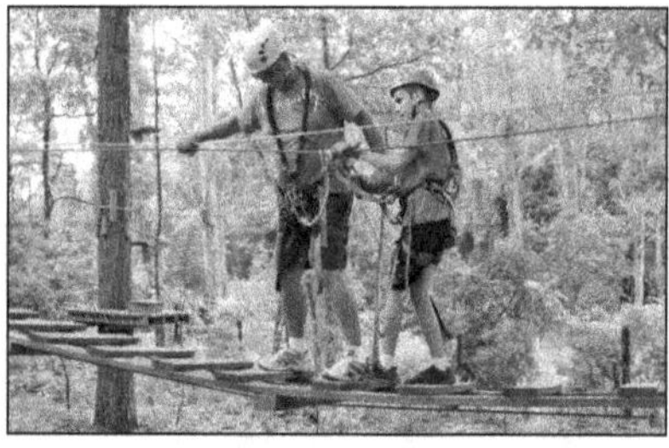

As a young boy and a young family, Sam and all of us have lost so much due to the hand that Mother Nature dealt him. However, we accepted that is how it was. We have never done the "The world owes us", "Woe is us" thing. There are so many people in the world who are far worse off than us and people struggling with unbelievable hardship every day. What happened to Sam and us does not mean that we put our hand out for compensation for our raw deal.

But in the next breath, I must say that Sam and our family have been unbelievably blessed to have been given opportunities beyond our wildest dreams. If I could have Sam with no cancer or vision impairment, I would be happy to not have had the adventures that he and we have had. But I am incredibly grateful to all of those individuals, associations and charities that have helped us struggle through the dark times and made it a little easier and a lot happier.

We were told about the different charities related to Sam's situation very early on in the diagnosis and treatment stage. However, as a very young baby, who was still going through a gruelling hospital regime, we didn't connect with any of the charities back then. It was only after a lot of his treatment had slowed down or stopped altogether that we became involved. Since then we have never looked back. Today, we are still having amazing adventures offered to us.

Starlight Children's Foundation

What an amazing charity organisation Starlight Children's Foundation is. We have had a huge variety of 'Escapes' and amazing experiences through them. We have been on family days out, going to places such as Healesville Sanctuary, The Melbourne Aquarium, Scienceworks, Circus Quirkus, Puffing Billy and the list goes on.

We have shared a family Christmas lunch with other 'Starlight' families at Vlado's Charcoal Grill in Richmond, Victoria. This is an annual Christmas lunch that Vlado Gregurek, and now his family, have been hosting for Starlight families for a number of years. Not only did we enjoy delicious food, which my mouth waters now just thinking about, but entertainment from some talented and giving Melbourne celebrities. And of course the day would not be complete without a visit from Humphrey B Bear and the fat man himself, Santa.

We have had family weekends/weeks away thanks to Starlight. We have been to Phillip Island to experience some of the local attractions and Beechworth for a relaxing week away just before Caitlin was born. These were wonderful opportunities, as they are getaways we would normally not be able to do. We were given the gift of time away as a family, without the stresses of home or hospital, which has been essential for our sanity.

Sam was asked to be on a Starlight donation 'Wish Card' brought out for the Christmas season in 2009. His photo was taken for the card and his and our story was put on the Starlight Children's Foundation website for people who had purchased a donation card to view. When we were asked to be part of this, we were honoured to be able to participate. For us, we have always been eager to give back if we could to those who have helped and supported us.

For 2013, Sam was awarded the honour of being named one of the '25 Year Ambassadors'. He was given a trophy at the Christmas luncheon at Vlado's to commemorate the honour.

Sam has been granted a 'Wish' from Starlight. As quoted on the Starlight website, "A Starlight Wish provides meaningful experiences, has life impacting benefits and is an opportunity to share in a dream come true. A Starlight Wish gives the whole family a break from the stress of their child's illness". As we have a number of years to be able to have Sam decide on his wish, he has not yet chosen what it will be. We would like him to make it meaningful and memorable, rather than just a big box of lollies, as a thirteen-year-old might choose!

And then there is the Starlight Express Room and the 'Captains'. Not only have we benefitted from these services, but so do children every day in hospitals throughout Australia. Seen as a 'haven inside the hospital', the Starlight Express Room "is a place where Captain Starlight orchestrates their own brand of fun and mayhem, alongside the latest computer games, movies, crafts and activities". The Starlight Express Room in the RCH helped us survive the worst day of our lives as parents, grandparents and family. Let me take you back to the day of Sam's second eye removal. We had come to the hospital that day as a family – myself, Sam, Jim, Mitchell, four grandparents, Jim's brother and his wife and their son. After waiting in the theatre waiting area, we decided we needed to take our mind off the reason we were there. Armed with a pager from the theatre waiting room, to tell us when to get back, we headed down to the Starlight Express Room. As we walked in there as a family, the atmosphere changed from doom and gloom to fun and excitement. We were greeted at the door by Captain Starlight, and after telling the Captain why we were there, the impromptu party began. Before we knew what was going on, we were all singing and dancing, my dad dancing with Captain Starlight. We were having a great time to see off Sam's sight. We still knew why we were at the hospital that day, but it made the waiting a little easier and happier.

And finally, last but not least, Captain Starlight. The Starlight website states that "Captain Starlight is a superhero from Planet Starlight, who transforms the hospital experience of children and young people, and their families across Australia. Captain Starlight is central to the fun, joy and laughter of the hospital experience. Captain Starlight provides distraction from the pain and stress of illness and its treatment, and while impact and transformation is immediate, it also has the longer term outcome of maintaining a strong sense of the individual and ensures their hospital experience is more positive".

Even just the other day, it was all shown to me what Captain Starlight does for and means to sick kids. I was waiting in the Monash Medical Centre for an outpatient appointment for our youngest, Caitlin. There was a dad there with his two daughters also waiting for an appointment. One of his daughters looked to have severe and multiple disabilities and was probably only five or six years old. Captain Starlight was entertaining the kids in the waiting room by making balloon animals, swords and flowers. He created a pretty flower for this young girl. When Captain Starlight handed her the flower and helped her hand to hold it, a big smile came over the girl's face. The dad looked at Captain Starlight and said "You're a life saver". And that's exactly what Captain Starlight is.

For everything, Starlight Children's Foundation, we thank you.

Camp Quality

Camp Quality's slogan is that "Laughter is the best medicine", and they definitely deliver on that. We have been to fun family days, to places near and far. We have been Ten Pin Bowling, to the Royal Melbourne Zoo, Luna Park, movies in the Royal Botanical Gardens, to the snow at Lake Mountain, Gumbuya Park, just to name a few.

We've been lucky to have been invited away on Family camps. With other families, we have stayed at farms, historic buildings, the beach and the snow. The family camps are an amazing time with our family and others. And the accidental counselling sessions that start with other parents in a relaxed, safe and understanding environment, are an added bonus. The Camp Quality volunteers are there to impose only two real rules – that we all have fun and that the parents relax. Very easy to get used to.

We have been to many Christmas parties at all kinds of venues – Luna Park, Adventure Park, Funfields, outdoor movies, Scienceworks, Campbelltown Miniature Railway, and more.

And our boys have also been on camps away from home, starting from the age of four. When any other parent may freak out at the thought of their child going off to a camp so young, it has been one of the most amazing things that Sam and Mitchell could have done. When the boys go to camp, they are paired up with a camp companion. This is one of the incredible CQ volunteers that are individually paired up with a child for the duration of the camp. And with our kids, I take my hat off to the companions that they have both had in past camps. You see, our boys are not ones to sit back and let the action happen around them. They get into everything that the camp experience has to offer, which means their companion does too. And although Sam is blind, it hasn't stopped him doing things on camp like riding a flying fox, doing a high ropes course or surfing.

One of the best things I have found with Camp Quality is that we have made some great connections and friends through all the activities. Not only have we connected with other families who know what each other go through, but we have made wonderful friends with many of the volunteers. They have become like an extended family to us, as they have seen all our children grow up along the way.

Thank you to our CQ family.

Challenge

Challenge is an amazing group. Sam's first experience with them was a camp at the age of six years old. This was the 'Cops & Kids' camp in Ballarat. We didn't quite know how he would be, first time away from home that wasn't at the grandparents. We had to pick up Sam early from the campsite at Sovereign Hill Ballarat, due to a hospital appointment. We thought he would run and cling to us. Well, weren't we sorely mistaken. He was too busy having fun and being angry at us that he had to leave early from the camp. He had an amazing time at the camp, doing everything at the Junior Camp (four to eight years old) including riding in a police car, a firetruck, and a tow truck, where he scared the driver when his prosthetic eye fell out. He went to a fire station, an indoor play centre, an airport and many other activities. They certainly don't just let the children sit back and watch life go by, they give the kids life changing experiences that money can't buy.

The boys have both been on camps with Challenge, Mitchell on the Junior Camps and Sam on the Junior and Urban Camps (eight to twelve years old). On Urban camp, Sam has been to the Royal Melbourne Show, spent a night sleeping under dinosaurs in the Melbourne Museum, visiting the Royal Melbourne Zoo, plus doing lots of activities and playing games. All of this with the wonderful help and support of his individual companion.

But Challenge has also taken care of Jim and myself. I have been lucky to have gone away for the weekend with half a dozen or so others mums on a 'Mums Retreat' weekend at Trevor Barker House, Torquay. Two beautiful ladies from Challenge took us down to the house, pampered us with a spa treatment, shopping, a chef-cooked meal at the house, wine, conversation and great company. We had the opportunity to talk about our families, our hospital journeys with our kids, or simply just chill out away from the problems of having a child with cancer.

I have also attended a lunch for Challenge mums in my area. A great chance for us mums to catch up with old friends and new to find out how all our kids are doing.

And the dads don't miss out either. Jim has had two separate weekends away with the Challenge DUC (Dads Ultimate Challenge) Club. He was able to go away with other dads who were also travelling the cancer journey. They were able to come together in an informal setting, participating in different activities and just doing 'blokey' things. I think Jim was a little worried it would be all 'sitting around in a circle, sharing feelings and singing Kumbaya', which of course it turned out not to be. He had a wonderful time away and met some other great dads, some who were still doing the cancer journey, and some who had been there and were now supporting others going through what they had.

And of course, there are the family day activities, including a Pirate adventure on boats off Williamstown, movie screenings, 'Taste of Melbourne' culinary experiences, and much more.

Then there's the huge Christmas party. A massive day at Sandown Racecourse, with carnival rides, petting zoo, endless amount of food, activities, and the special event for the big kids as much as the little ones – the hot-rod and Harley rides. And of course, a visit from Santa.

Thank you for everything Challenge. Keep doing what you do so well, you make such a difference to all of our lives.

Ronald McDonald House Family Retreats

We have experienced the relaxation of visiting a few Ronald McDonald beach houses both in Victoria and New South Wales. The Ronald McDonald House Charities created the Ronald McDonald Family Retreats to help relieve the burden of immense emotional, physical and financial stress that families of children experiencing a serious illness are often placed under. They offer a place for families with a seriously ill child to enjoy a holiday together, take a break from the stresses of hospital and deal with their new life situation.

We have been able to have quality time away together to Kessia's Cottage at Ocean Grove, Victoria; Fiona Lodge at Bateman's Bay, NSW; a Ronald

McDonald Beach House property at Forster, NSW; and the Family Retreat House in Bunbury, WA. All of these have provided an amazing family holiday away, time together that, with day to day life, is sometimes hard to prioritise. We are eternally grateful for these opportunities for a family break, which wouldn't happen otherwise.

The above charities who have helped us have given us more than dollars could ever buy. They have given us the opportunities to spend time as a family, without the stress of having a sick or disabled child who is unable to participate in activities with us. They have given Sam the possibility of doing things that would be otherwise out of reach to him. They have treated him as a 'normal' kid, not a sick or disabled one. They have also given Mitchell, and now Caitlin, opportunities as the sibling of a 'cancer kid' that would normally not be available to them. As the sibling of a child going through a life threatening illness or hospital treatment, they may get left behind, their needs put on the backburner while the entire family's life is put on hold for the needs of the sick child. These amazing organisations realise that this could be a huge problem, and address it accordingly. They are made to feel important and valued, not left behind.

After being immersed into the world of these amazing charities and the incredible people who both work and volunteer for them, as a parent I cannot tell you how invaluable their support is. Whenever the opportunity arises to be able to help and support them, please do so. The difference they make to families cannot be put into words.

Again, as a family, we thank you.

Sam's
day with
W.E.S.T.
2007

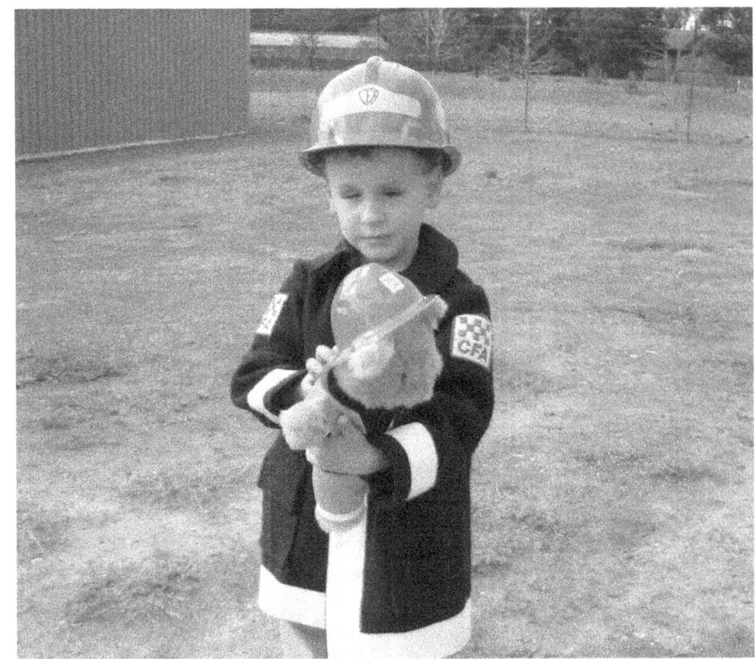

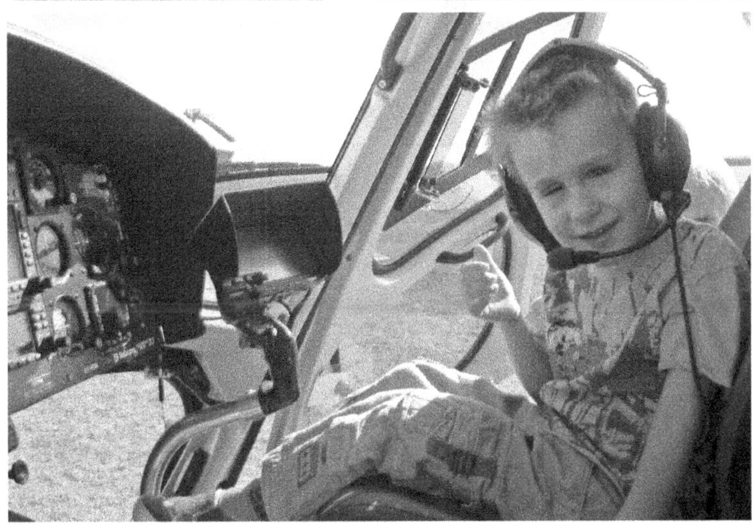

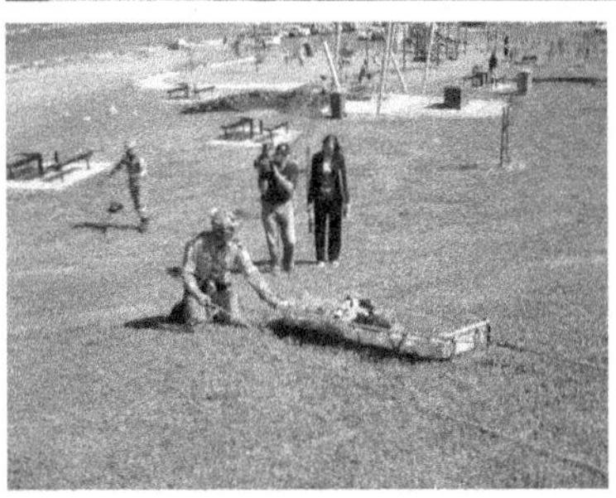

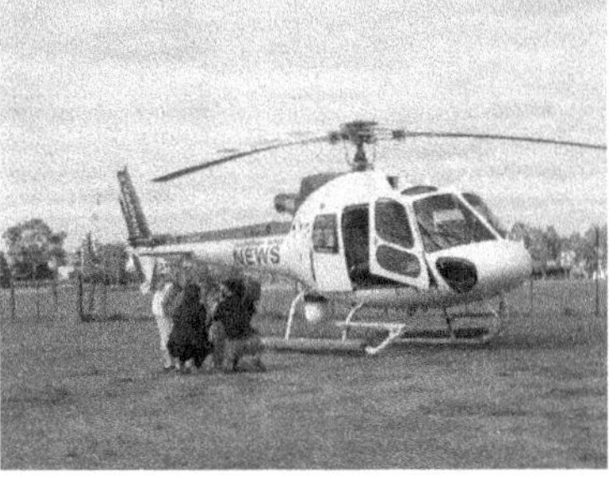

Sam's amazing adventures in Disneyland and Hollywood 2007

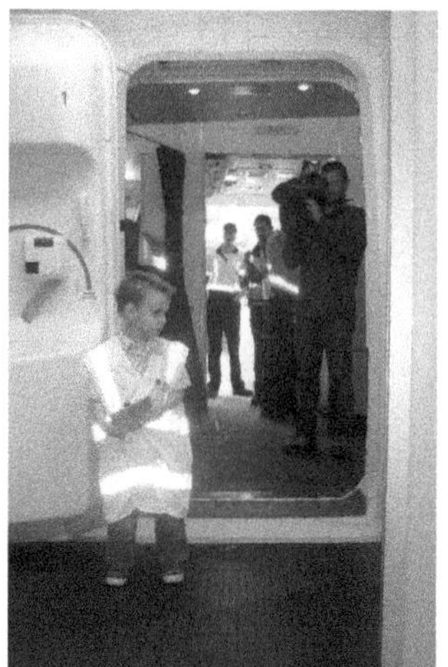

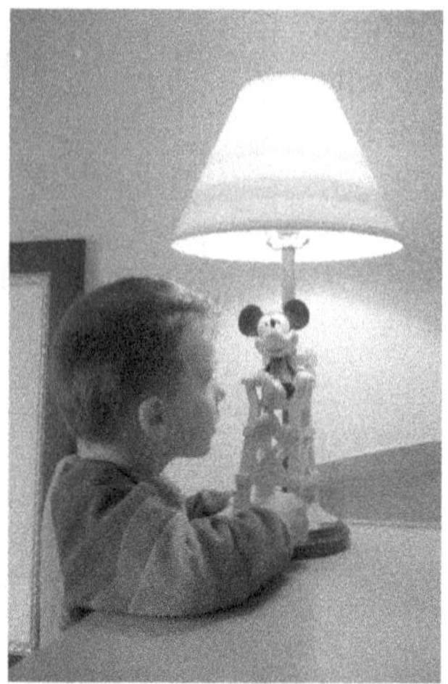

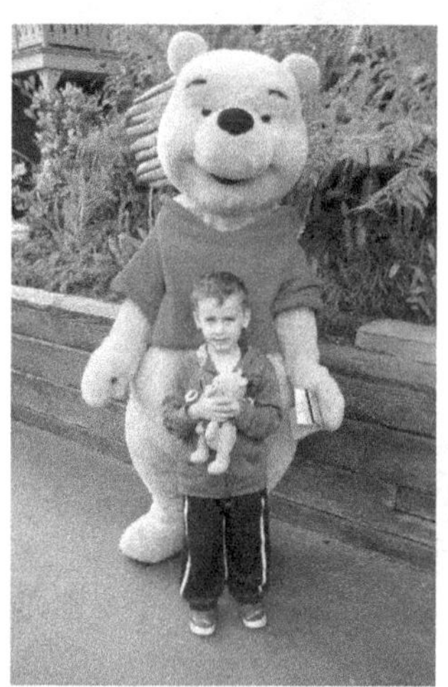

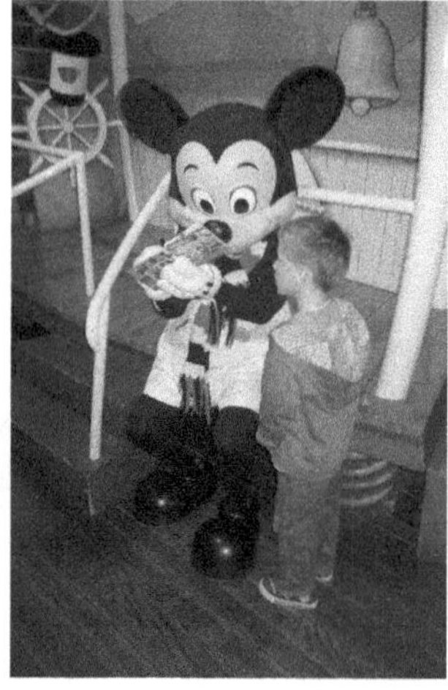

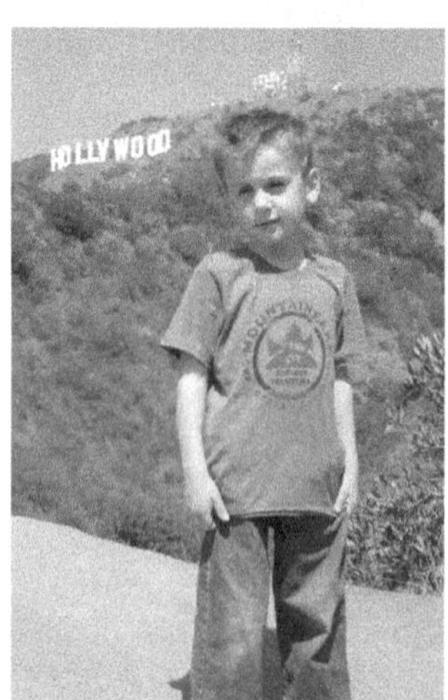

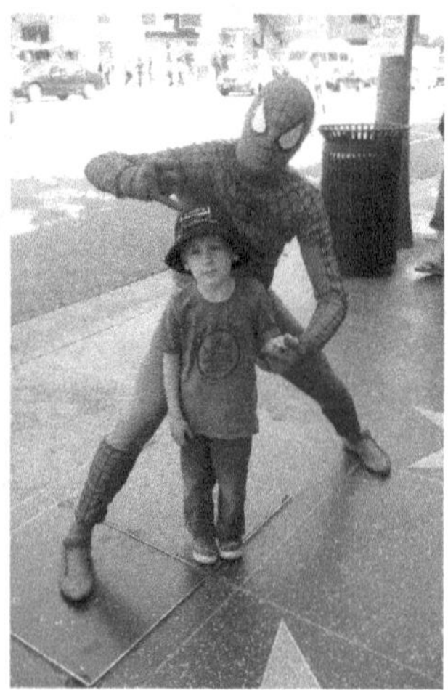

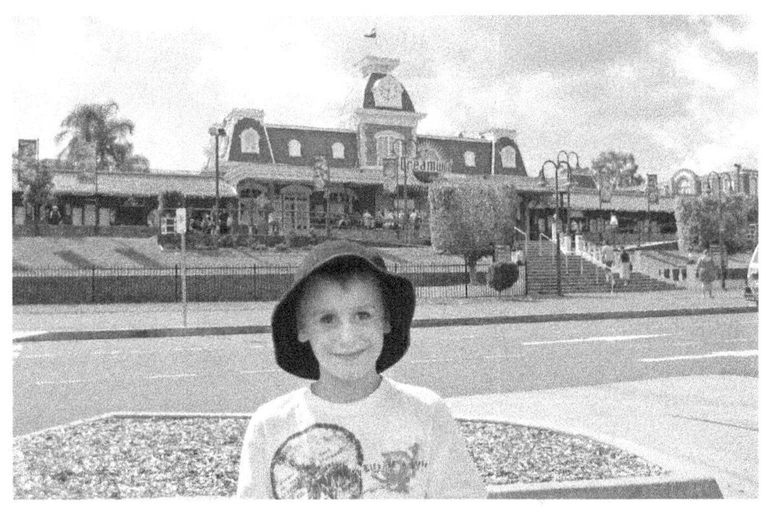

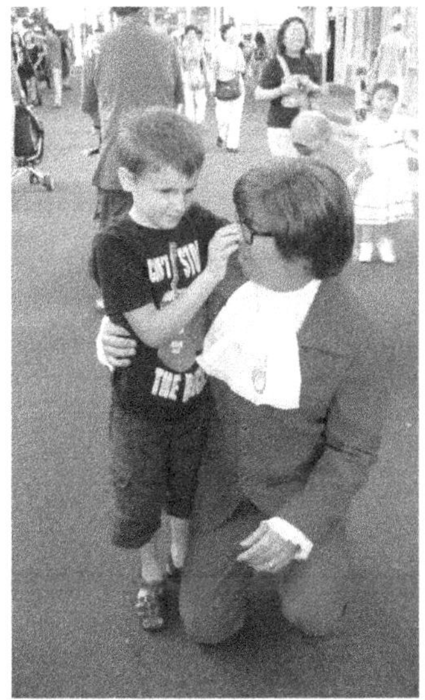

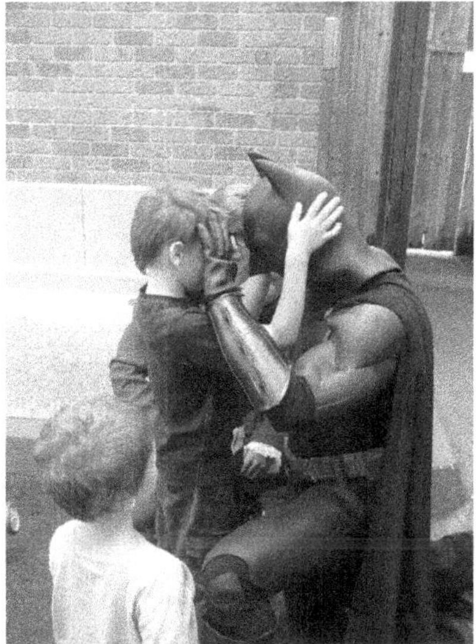

Theme Park fun on the Gold Coast 2010

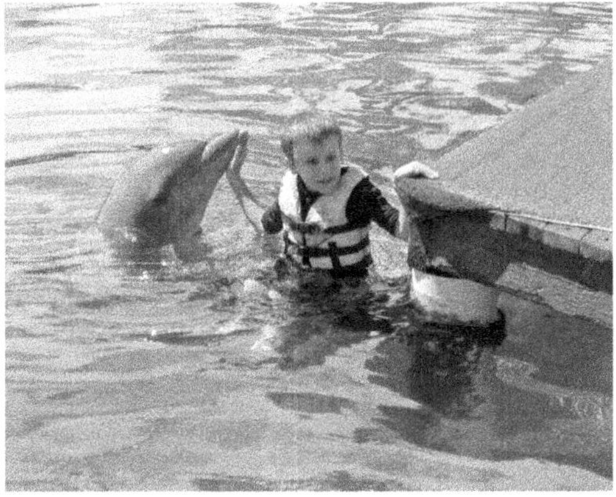

Beyond Sight Family Fun Day 2007

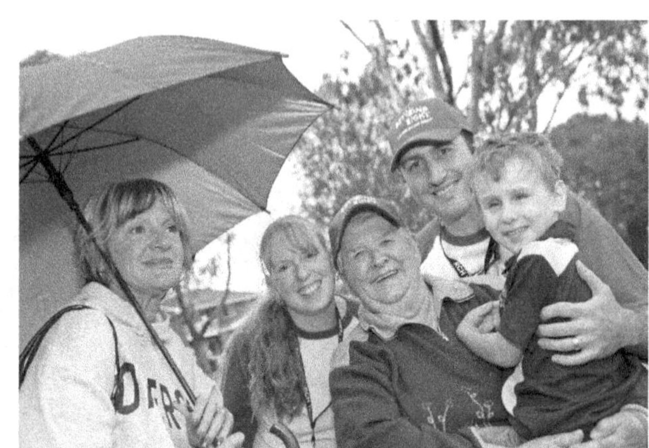

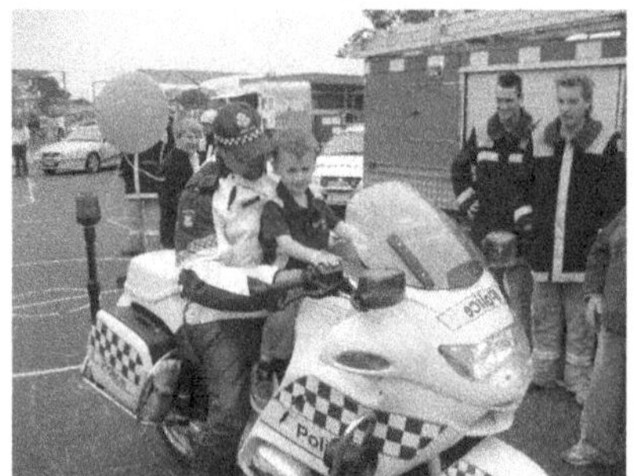

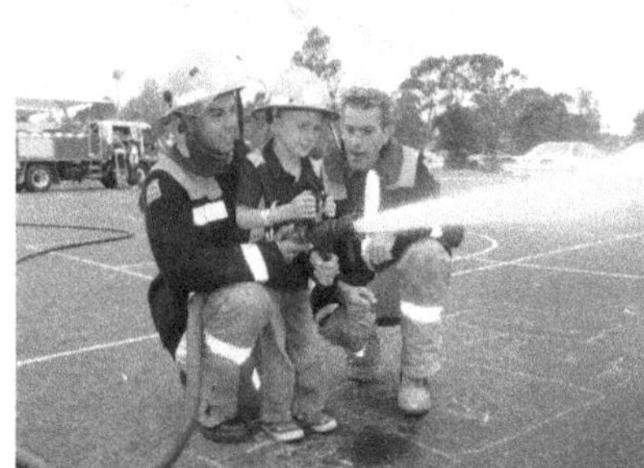

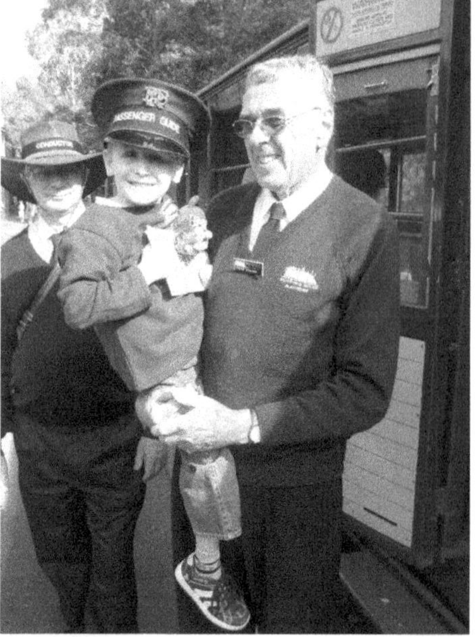

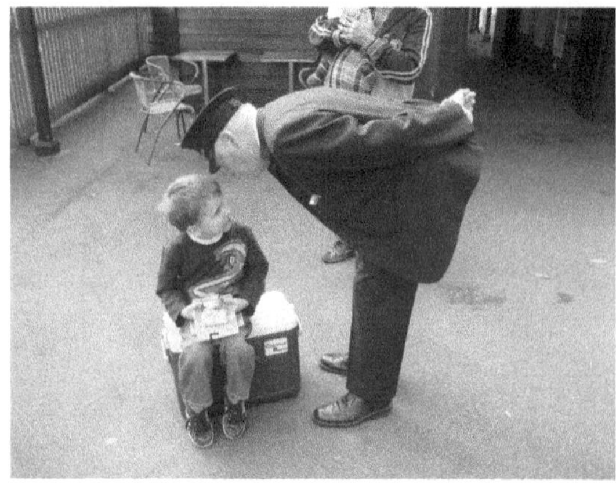

Puffing Billy 2007

The day that changed our lives 2007

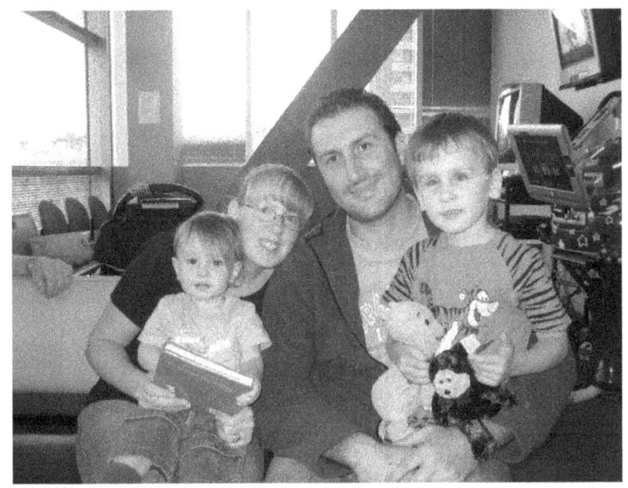

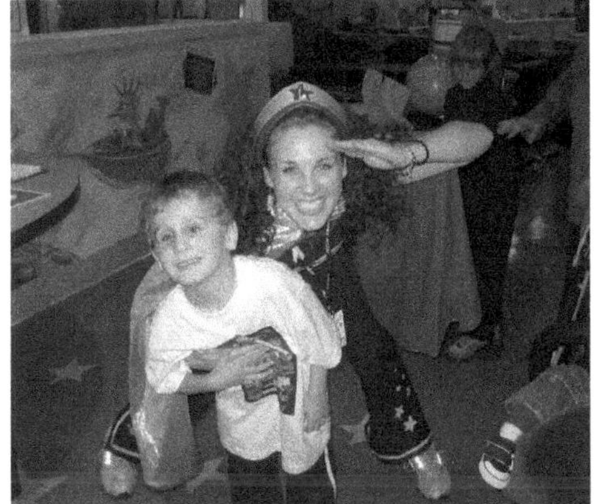

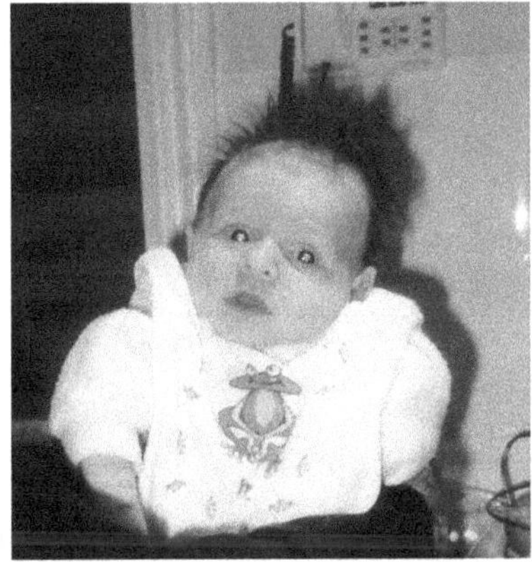

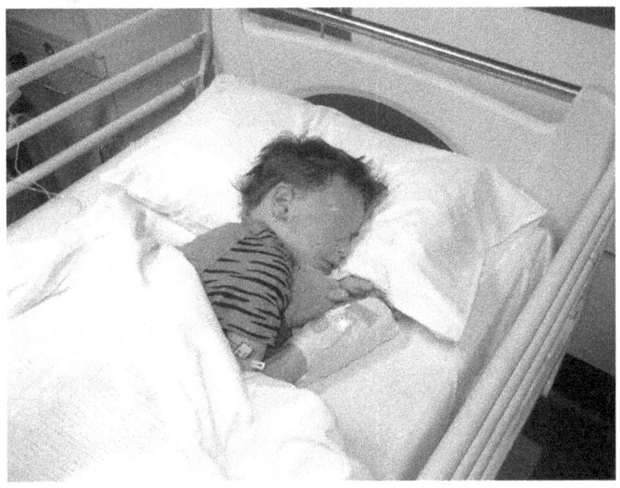

Some of the amazing people (and bears) we've met along the way

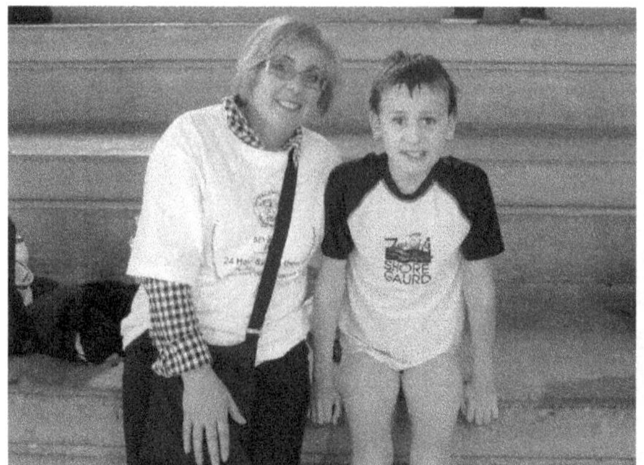

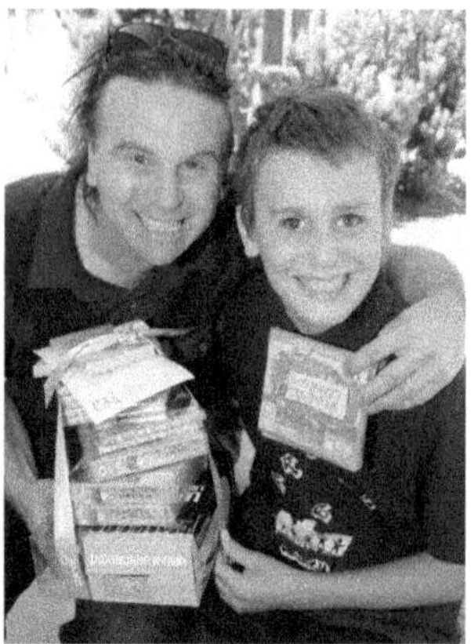

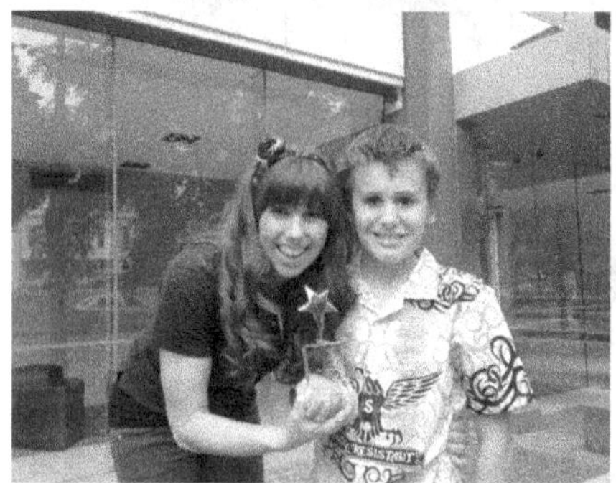

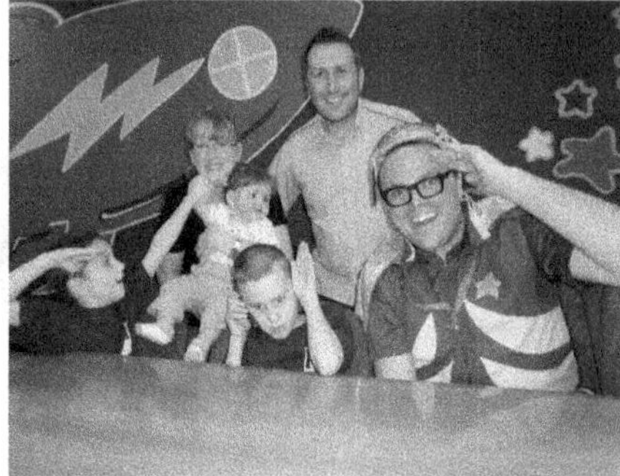

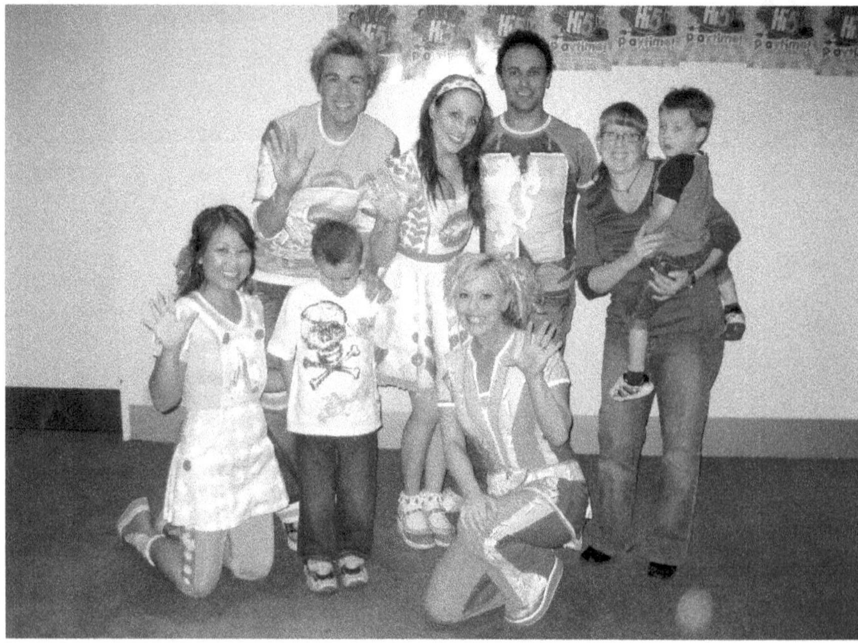

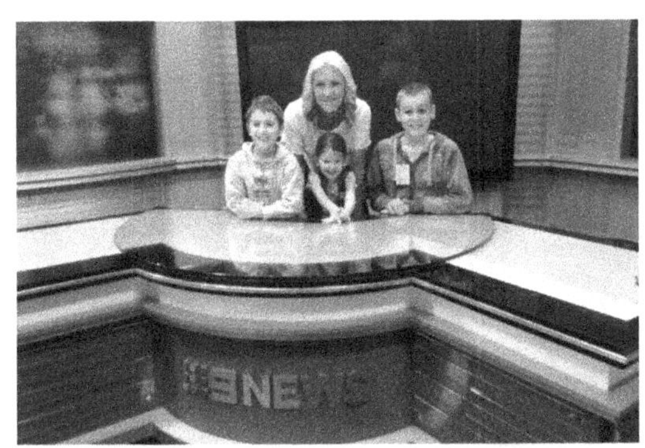

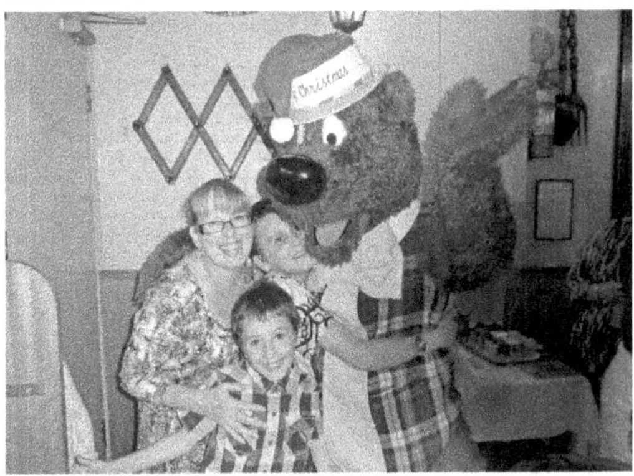
Christmas

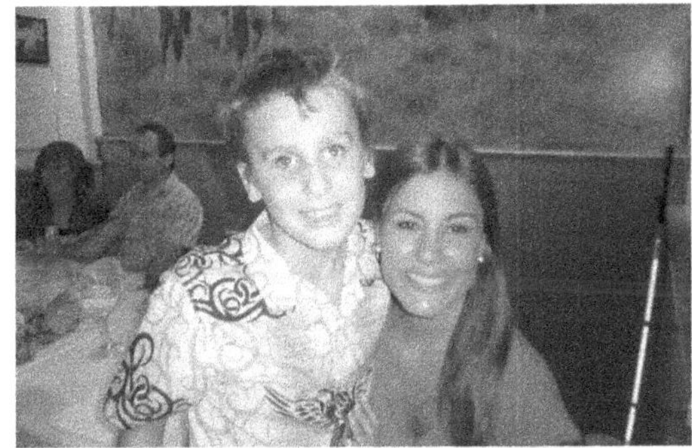

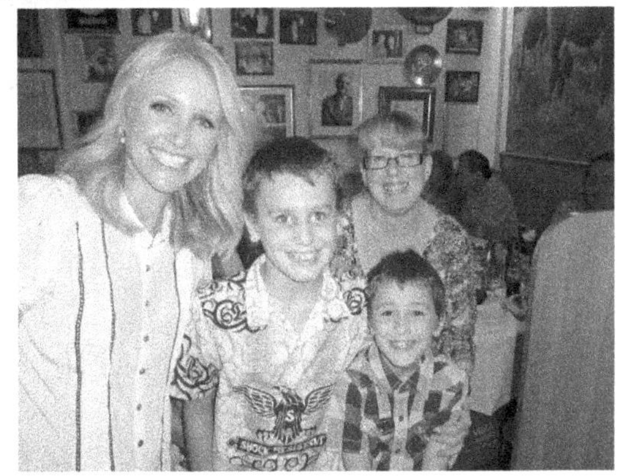

Family is everything

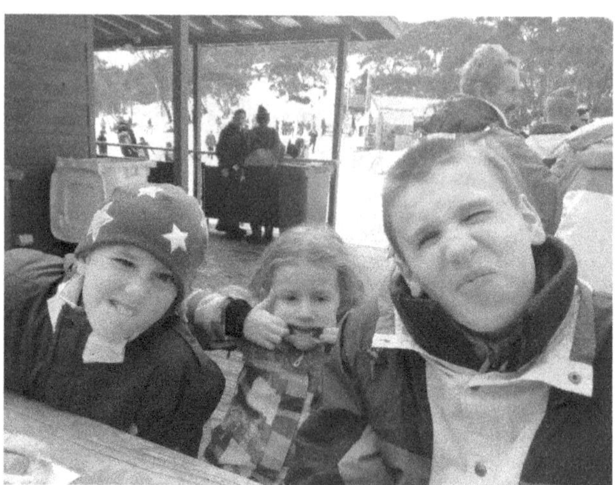

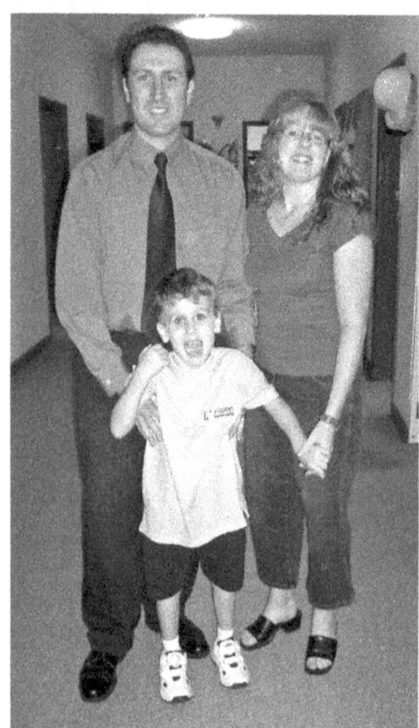

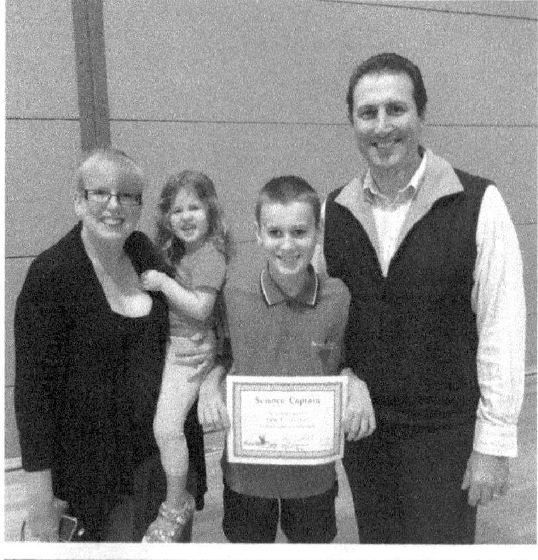

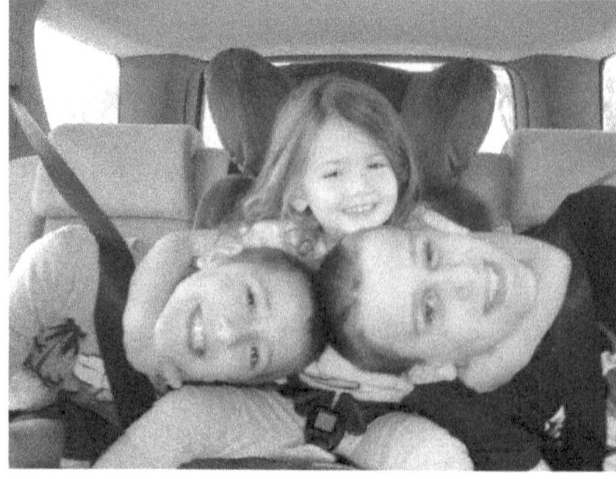

...and then there was Sam

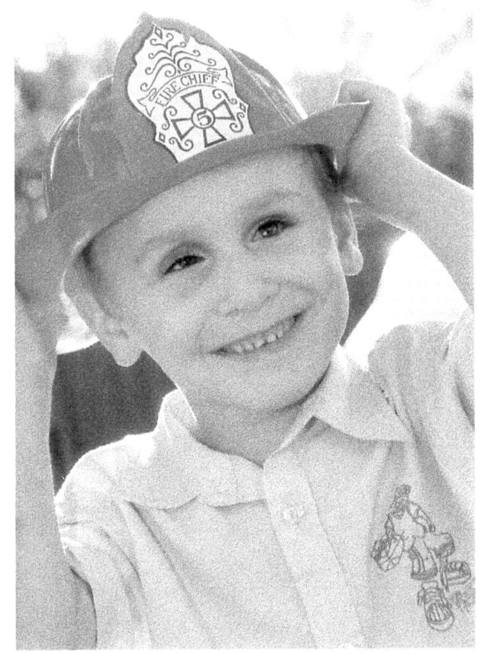

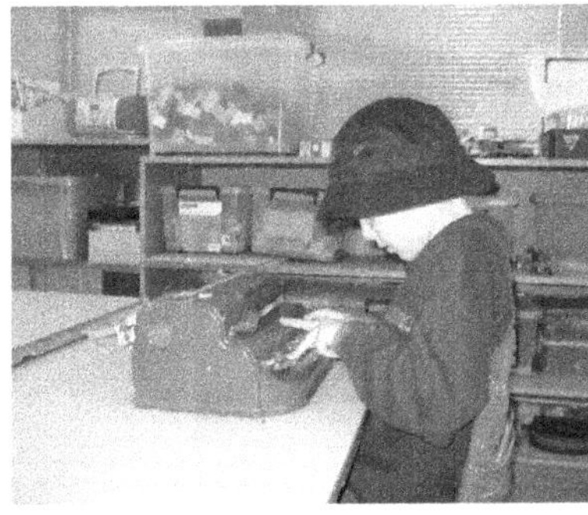

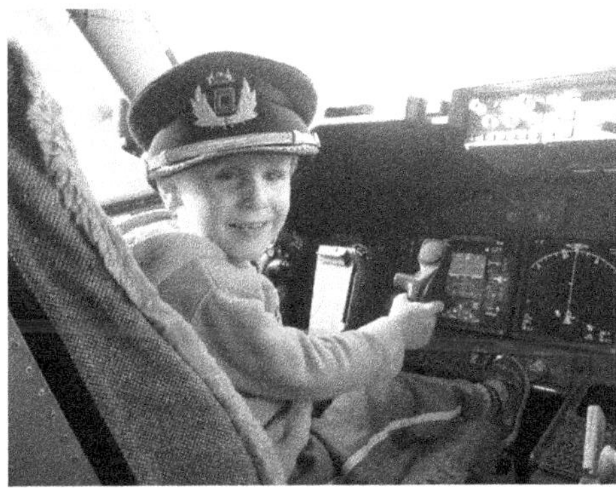

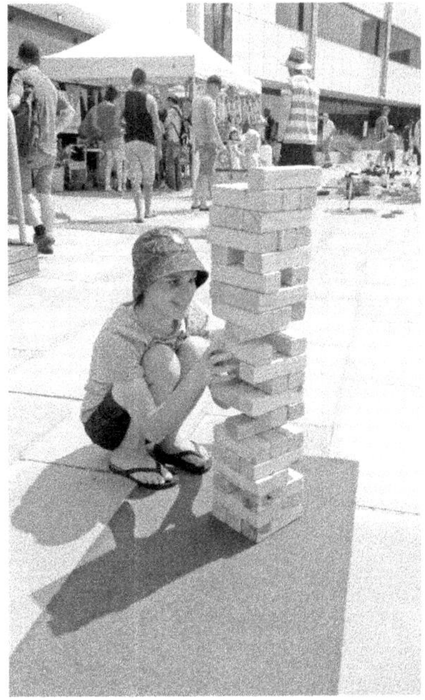

CHAPTER 10

A DAY (OR TWO) TO REMEMBER

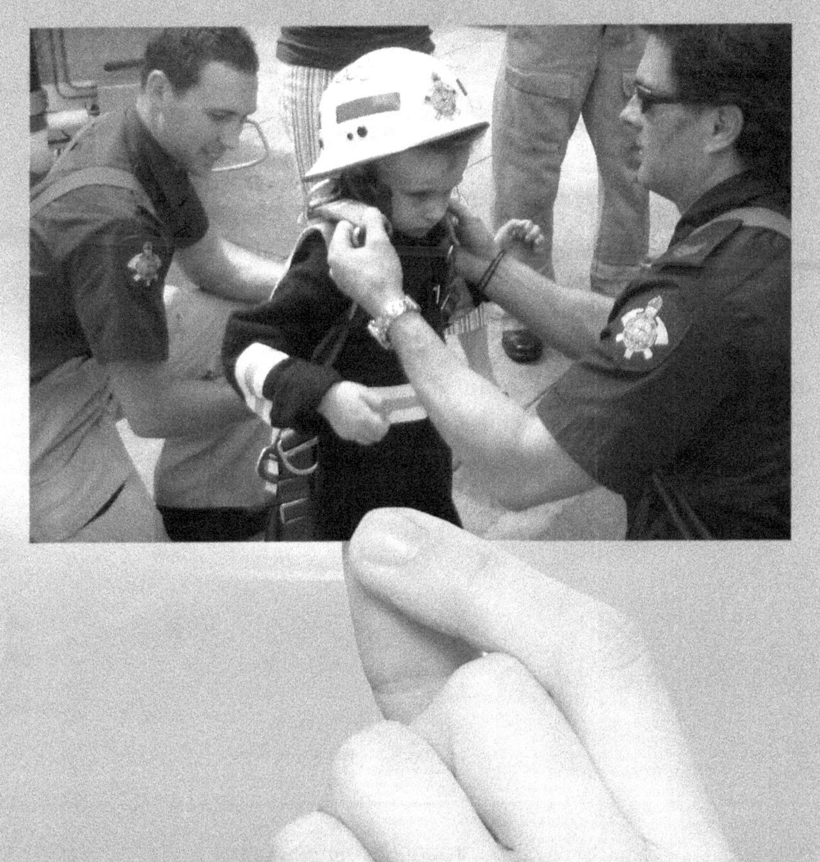

Chapter 10

A Day (Or Two) To Remember

(Jim)

Move Aside, Make Way, for Fireman Sam

Fireman Sam – Created by Rob Lee
HIT Entertainment Company

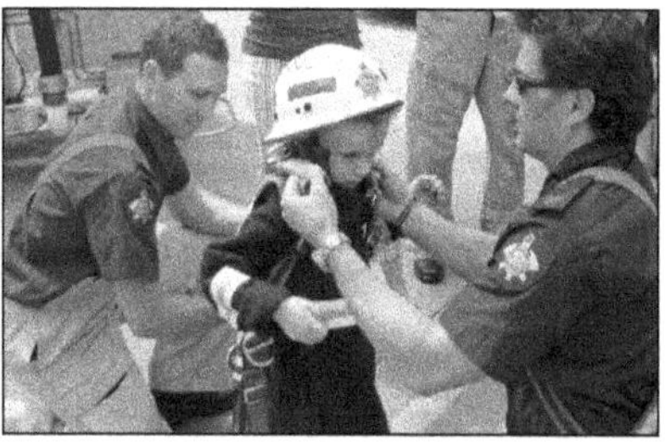

As parents, all you want for your children is health and happiness. Unfortunately, we didn't have full control over Sam's health, but we could certainly have an influence on his happiness.

At the height of his intensive treatment we were keen to give Sam as many memorable experiences as possible to keep his spirits up. During this period, he was very much into Fireman Sam, especially since he shared his name with the lead character.

Eastern Hill Fire Station 1

Lisa took a punt and contacted the MFB (Metropolitan Fire Brigade) Headquarters in East Melbourne. She was lucky enough to speak to the right person, who was touched by our story. We were hoping to organise a quick visit to one of the fire stations, but it worked out to be so much more than that. It was going to be a full on experience with all the 'bells and whistles'.

The date was set and we were invited down to Fire Station 1 at Eastern Hill. We even had a special Fireman Sam T-shirt made for Sam to mark the occasion. I took the day off work because this was something that I definitely wanted to share with him. After all, what little boy doesn't want to grow up to be a Fireman!

From the moment we arrived they made us feel very welcome. We were introduced to some office staff and then greeted by two young firefighters named Conan and Daniel, who would accompany us around the Fire Station and fully immerse Sam in the experience they had planned.

Sam was given a fireman's uniform to wear, complete with helmet and a name badge naming him as an Honorary Firefighter for the day. He also received a very special teddy bear dressed up as a fireman, which he aptly named 'Terry' after one of the Station Officers on duty.

We were taken out into the station and shown around. Sam was given the VIP treatment with unrestricted access to all the areas. He was able to look at one of the fire engines including the equipment storage compartments, extend a high rise ladder, put on the breathing apparatus, go into the mobile command centre, use a fire hose and fire extinguisher and slide down the fireman's pole. Wow, what an experience for a four-and-a-half-year-old!

It was then time for the real treat of the day... to go out in one of the fire engines around the city streets with lights flashing and sirens blaring. Sam got to hold one of the walkie-talkies as they set up a mock emergency. He had a big grin on his face from ear to ear as he soaked it all up.

The fun didn't stop there. When we got back to the station Sam was then harnessed into a cherry picker (aka a snorkel) with Lisa and raised up to the rooftop of the building. I was fortunate enough to see it all from up above. I think he finally realised that this is not the sort of thing that happens every day to children his age. The MFB went above and beyond for our family that day and we will be forever grateful.

Once all the planned activities had finished, we were taken for a guided tour through the station and even got to see the private quarters and mess hall. Sam had a quick game of table tennis with the Firefighters that were on standby, which he really enjoyed.

At the end of the day we were offered a large platter of food and got to relive our experience with the staff over a casual lunch. A few weeks later we received a fully edited DVD of the whole event, which Sam will still watch now from time to time. Thank you to a very special group of people who put their lives on the line to help, serve and protect others.

Western Emergency Services Team (W.E.S.T)

On a beautiful autumn day in March 2007, we were invited out to the Western Bulldogs Community Festival and Family Day at the Whitten Oval. We had been in and out of the media around that time and had people contacting us to see if there was anything that they could do for Sam or our family, as we were promoting a Family Fun Day to raise funds and awareness for retinoblastoma. Lisa and Sam were interviewed live on air by one of the local radio stations at this event.

During this period, we came across Sergeant Ron, who felt a deep connection with Sam and his plight. As we had been given a date by the doctors at the RCH when he would lose his sight by having his remaining eye removed, Ron wanted to do something that would remain in Sam's memory bank for life. The Western Emergency Services Team (W.E.S.T.) had planned to involve the whole team to do their small part and bring the whole day together into one big extravaganza.

We were asked to meet the Channel 9 News helicopter out at the Moorabbin Airport on the 18th March 2007. Lisa and Sam were nervously excited to be flown from the South Eastern suburbs of Melbourne to the West, while I drove our car to meet them at the Werribee Police Station. They were greeted by a team of emergency services staff, some friends from hospital and a Channel 9 News reporter with a cameraman, who followed us around and compiled a story for the evening news that night. He was changed into a junior firefighter's outfit and kindly handed another teddy bear. We built up a small collection of furry friends during this time and he enjoyed having them around to comfort him.

The Western Emergency Services Team is made up of the Victoria Police, Country Fire Authority (CFA), State Emergency Service (SES) and Coast Guard. They had all their vehicles lined up for Sam to explore, which is exactly what he did. Sam has always been a very curious boy and that is what I believe will get him far in life.

The next part of the adventure was a ride in one of the police vehicles to the Werribee Fire Station. He was then taken aboard one of the fire rescue vehicles and shown where all of the equipment is stored in time of need. He was loaded up into the cabin and got to turn the sirens on. What boy doesn't like to test the sirens? I was fortunate enough to accompany him for the second leg of our journey in the fire engine to the mouth of the Werribee River.

This is where the SES took charge of the operation and performed a mock rescue on Sam, who they strapped into a stretcher and brought him down the hill using guide ropes. He couldn't quite understand what was going on, but he just went along with it.

From there he was walked down to the jetty hand in hand by Sergeant Ron and Mark from the CFA, where an SES inflatable rubber dinghy was waiting to take him out into the bay. He was fitted with a life vest and taken for a quick spin. Luckily it wasn't too choppy!

It was then onto the home stretch, which saw him jump aboard the Coast Guard. Lisa suffers from hydrophobia, so I was given permission to join Sam on the cruise on Port Phillip Bay back to Williamstown. He explored every square inch of the boat and even got to sit at the controls for a while. He enjoyed the wind blowing through his hair and watching the wake behind the boat.

When we finally arrived at Williamstown everybody was there waiting for us with opens arms. This was the end of our big adventure but certainly not one that would be forgotten in a hurry. By that stage Sam was starving, so he had some lunch and then we said our goodbyes. We finished off the day by going into the Williamstown Police Station and telling the staff in there what a great day we had.

It is difficult to put into words what that day meant to us as a family, but more importantly Sam who was made to feel incredibly special. The human spirit is still alive and well!

CHAPTER 11

SAM'S AMAZING ADVENTURES

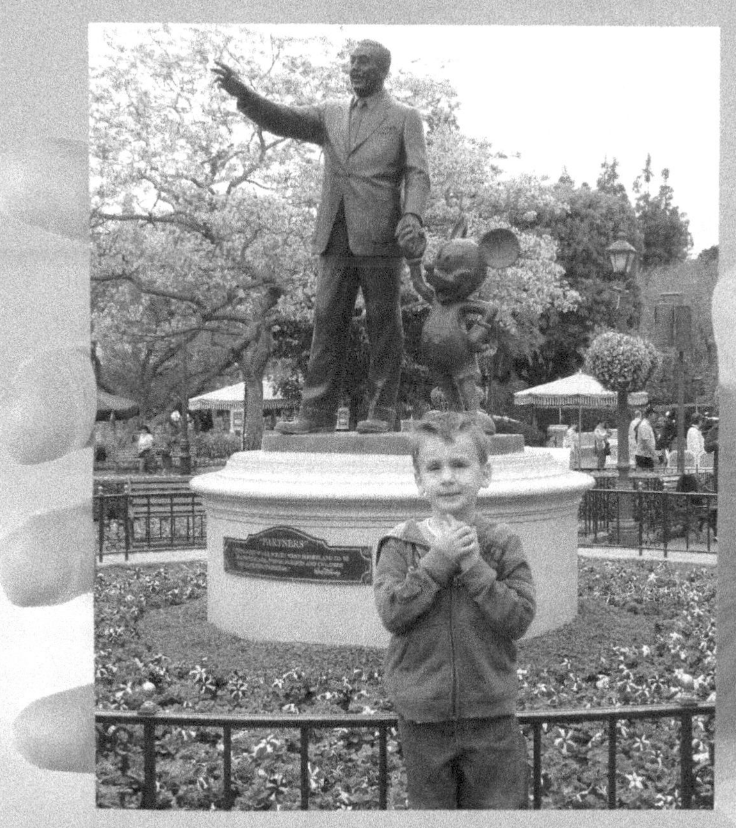

Chapter 11

Sam's Amazing Adventures

(Jim)

If you can dream it, you can do it.

Walt Disney

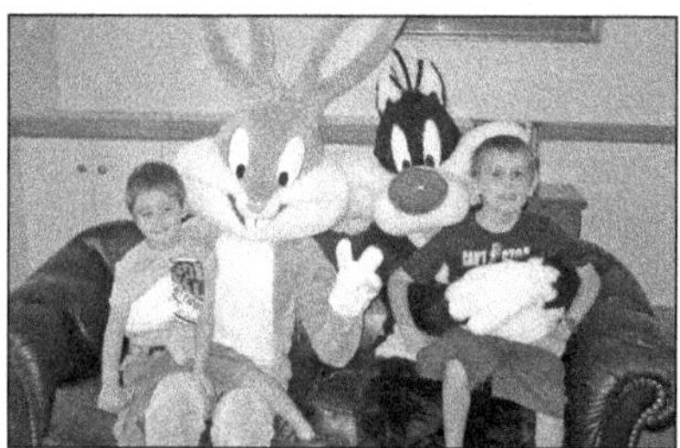

As difficult as our journey has been as a family, there have also been some amazing opportunities and experiences that we have been a part of, which has helped distract us from the battles that we have had to endure. We are eternally grateful to the people and organisations who bring joy and light to the lives of others that may have an illness or are less fortunate.

We made it our mission as parents, once we were told Sam would be made totally blind, to give him as many visual memories as possible which he could experience and remember forever.

There are far too many adventures to share, but these are the main ones that stand out in Sam's mind and he likes to relive.

Disneyland

At the height of our battle to save Sam's sight in 2006, we received a call out of the blue from Channel 9. They asked us to make ourselves available later in the week for a car that would pick us up and drive us into the Bourke Street Mall, where *The Today Show* was filming for the Melbourne Cup Carnival. We had no idea what this was all about and it had our minds racing, trying to come up with a million different scenarios of how it would all play out.

When we arrived into the city, Lisa, Samuel and myself were escorted up the mall where we waited for our cue. We could see the hosts and crew of *The Today Show* recording the show and got all excited with what was potentially to come. We only thought we were there to watch a live recording of the show or a meet and greet at best.

Then we were approached by one of the floor crew and asked to mic up as we were about to be introduced onto the show, which went national, and were going to be interviewed by the two hosts, Karl Stefanovic and Jessica Rowe. My heart started to pound and the nerves came over me. What was this all about?

The countdown began as they came out of an ad break... Three, Two, One. We were on live national TV with Sam in my arms and right on cue he started crying and screaming uncontrollably trying to escape from my clutches. Lisa as per usual, took control of the situation and shared our experience of Sam's battle with the audience. They wanted to know about our story and how Sam was doing with his treatment.

We then had another gentleman come onto the set and introduce himself as a representative from Travelscene. *The Today Show* had apparently received a letter from our neighbour's Rebecca and Brendan for their 'Week of Wishes', outlining our story and the fact that Sam may be losing his sight in the not too distant future.

He then went on to say that they were going to send our young family of four on an all-expenses paid holiday to Disneyland in Anaheim, America, to make some happy memories for Sam and us. We were both shocked and dumbfounded and didn't know what to say apart from "Thank you, thank you, thank you." I said a few words on camera, but it was all a blur.

We went to 'The Happiest Place on Earth' during our honeymoon in 1999 and had always vowed to return with our kids when they were old enough, but hoping it would be under very different circumstances.

From the moment we found out that we were heading to Disneyland, it was a bit of a whirlwind and we couldn't contain our excitement. We had to organise passports for the kids and work out a suitable time when we could go in amongst all the hospital visits. We eventually booked the trip in for April 2007, a month before the inevitable operation to remove Sam's remaining eye.

We received many messages of support and well wishes during this period from family, friends and people we'd never even met. We were also contacted by QANTAS, with whom we were flying, to go in for a tour of the Melbourne Tullamarine Airport and the Boeing 747 Jumbo we would be taking over to America, the day before our departure.

We had an early morning meeting with a Channel 9 news reporter at the Airport, as the public had taken an interest in Sam's story and they wanted to follow it through to the end.

We were greeted by Jane in Marketing/PR and 'Captain John' the Pilot for a behind the scenes tour of the airport, which the general public wouldn't normally get to see. We were made to feel very special.

We made our way through security and baggage handling where we were taken aboard the Jumbo Jet, which we had all to ourselves. We rushed through economy class to have a look at the meal preparation areas on board and then business class, but more than anything wanted to go upstairs to check out first class and the cockpit.

We were able to take our time looking around first class and sat down in the comfortable, lounge style seats while the reporter interviewed us. I think Sam was impressed, because Lisa and I certainly were. That's how we should all travel!!!

John then offered to take us into the cockpit where he explained how the controls work to make the plane fly and other stuff that went over our heads. He placed a pilot's hat on Sam's head and got him to sit down in the pilot's seat, which made him feel very important indeed.

We took our time getting off the plane, even though we were going to be on it again in less than 24 hours. It was all part of the big adventure and hopefully something that Sam would never forget.

At the end of the tour, John and Jane gave Sam a show bag full of goodies he could remember the day by and lock away in his memory bank. It did the trick, because to this day he still talks about the day he got to be an honorary pilot and have a Jumbo Jet all to himself!

The day had finally arrived when we would be leaving for the USA, bound for Disneyland and all it had to offer. We decided to stay on a little longer and visit Beverly Hills, Hollywood, Santa Monica and Venice Beach, because it's not every day you get to travel to the other side of the world.

We thought that having an overnight flight on such a long journey would be a good chance for the boys to get some sleep, but they had other ideas due to the fact that it was their first time flying. Mitchell was only 12 months old at the time and this was all a big adventure for him, so we were lucky to get an hour or two of sleep out of him, as it was more fun crawling up and down the aisles, into Business Class and in between the seats. Sam was full of adrenalin, so he had minimal shut-eye as well.

When we got to America, Lisa and I were both so exhausted and couldn't wait to get our luggage and make our way to the hotel which was located in

Anaheim. We caught a coach from LAX to Disney's Paradise Pier Hotel which was only a hop, skip and jump from Disneyland. I still remember Lisa vomiting into her jumper, because by now the lack of sleep had gotten to her, and she suffered from travel sickness at the best of times. The kids and I couldn't help but laugh… we all thought it was hilarious!

We checked in and made our way up to the room, which had great views out to the pool and water slide, that we didn't get a chance to use. We had a three or four-day pass to the two theme parks and wanted to make the most of it and spend every waking hour soaking it all in. With zero sleep and the jet lag not having kicked in yet, we decided to take the plunge and head straight over to Disneyland.

I can recall our first walk from the hotel along the promenade with the Disney music playing in the background over the loudspeakers and lots of families everywhere with big smiles on their faces as we approached the long queues.

We avoided the lengthy wait because we had prepaid tickets, and it just so happened to be one of the busiest weeks on the American calendar due to the Easter break. As we scanned our tickets and walked through the turnstiles a weird sensation came over me. It was a bittersweet moment and quite emotional, because we were finally here with our children, but this would be the last time that Sam would "see" this magical place.

There was so much going on and we didn't know where to look or what to do first. We decided the best thing to do was to make our way over to guest services and ask if there was anything that may be worthwhile doing for children with a visual impairment. They were very helpful and offered some suggestions and the two boys even came away with a stuffed toy each as gifts from Disneyland. They both still have Winnie the Pooh and Tigger in their toy collections.

We slowly worked our way around all the different worlds over the course of the time we were there and made sure that Sam met each of the Disney characters as we saw them, because it was so busy and we might not get another opportunity. It was very overwhelming for Sam and such a memorable experience, which we feel has fuelled his love of thrill rides to this day.

It has been called 'The Happiest Place on Earth' and for very good reason, because even the adults become children again and have so much fun there. All of your cares are forgotten and you fully immerse yourself in the whole experience. We will definitely have to take Mitchell back along with Caitlin, because he spent the bulk of his time sleeping in the pram.

The first time we went there on our honeymoon in 1999, California Adventure Park hadn't been built, let alone open, so it was good to explore. I think of it more like Disneyland for adults.

It now feels like a lifetime ago, yet the memories are still so vivid. We hired a car and drove from Anaheim to Los Angeles, which was an experience in itself. I've seen the Californian freeways on TV, but to actually drive on them is like taking your life into your own hands!

We stayed at the Crowne Plaza in Beverly Hills, which was like another world to us. When we weren't driving around we were using public transport. Sam has always loved catching the bus, train or tram and desperately wants his independence.

There was so much to see and do there and we certainly made the most of it. From Rodeo Drive to the La Brea Tar Pits, from the Hollywood Walk of Fame to Grauman's Chinese Theatre and up to the famous 'HOLLYWOOD' sign in the Hollywood Hills.

We also made a special trip down to the famous Santa Monica Pier that is home to Pacific Park amusement park and then over to Venice Beach, known for the Boardwalk and Muscle Beach Gym where they pump iron and you come across all kinds of weird and whacky individuals.

This was a once in a lifetime experience for our family and we will be eternally grateful that Sam was able to see the magical Disneyland as a child, because he lost his sight in less than a month after we returned. Sam had an absolute ball and he is waiting for the day when we can all return again, and this time it will also be with Caitlin. Thank you Walt for your foresight and vision.

The Gold Coast

In 2009 we moved into our new house in Berwick and earlier that year Sam had started Grade One at the newly opened Berwick Chase Primary School. There were a few articles written about our story in the local paper which caught people's attention.

Lisa was contacted shortly afterwards by Ron who lived in the area and was a committee member of the Noble Park Rotary Club. He invited us down to one of their meetings and dinner as his guest.

After dinner it was onto the order of business. To our surprise, Ron got up and started sharing our story with the room. Rotary are all about the community and their mission is to provide service to others. We were then informed that they were offering to send our family on an all-expenses paid holiday to the Gold Coast in Queensland and they would be honoured if we would accept. We could choose a suitable time to take it, so there was no rush to do it straight away.

It was a very humbling experience to say the least, and especially to know that there are wonderful people out there who are willing to bring joy to the lives of others that they don't even know. We were extremely grateful for the opportunity and couldn't wait to share our experience with them when we returned.

When we told Sam, he was jumping out of his skin with excitement. This time around Mitchell would be old enough to enjoy some of the rides and take in the whole experience, unlike the family trip we took to Disneyland years before when he spent most of the time sleeping in his pram.

It was an early morning start with the sparrows on the day of our flight in March 2010. We made our way to Tullamarine Airport and left our car in the multi-level long term car park which was closest to the terminals. Sam loves flying and would travel by plane anywhere and everywhere if he could. As a family, we tend to do a lot of driving holidays, much to his disgust.

A few hours later we made a safe landing at the Gold Coast Airport in Coolangatta. We decided to hire a car for the time that we were there as it would be a lot easier to get around with two young children. We made our way up to the Paradise Resort Hotel which was about 40 minutes away at Surfers Paradise. It was a family friendly hotel specifically designed with kids in mind. We couldn't have chosen a better place to stay as it had everything we needed and more.

We checked in and set ourselves up for the next ten days. We all had a look around the resort to get our bearings and whet the appetite for what was to come. They had a kids' club, games room, playgrounds, multiple pools, spa, poolside café and bar, BBQ area, a number of restaurants and minimart. We have since found out that they have now added a new waterpark and ice rink to top it off. It's heaven on earth for kids.

Because we had the freedom of a car we could come and go as we pleased. This gave us an opportunity to get out and about to explore some of the region such as Southport, Tamborine Mountain, Thunderbird Park and the Carrara Markets. It would've been good to see more, but we were there for one main reason and that was the Theme Parks!!!

The first cab off the rank was Dreamworld and the boys couldn't wait to get in there to cut loose. They got to meet lots of characters including The Wiggles favourites like Dorothy, Wags, Henry and Captain Feathersword, not to mention Dora the Explorer, SpongeBob and Patrick. There was fun around every corner and Sam being the adrenalin junkie, went on absolutely every ride. He has no fear, and why would you when you can't see the danger. It was an awesome experience.

We took a break from the Theme Parks for a day and went back to nature at the Currumbin Wildlife Sanctuary. We got to mix it with some of the local wildlife and the boys along with Lisa got to hold a cute koala and a baby crocodile, but avoided getting too close to the adult crocodiles. There were all kinds of birds, marsupials and reptiles which kept the boys entertained for the day. I tried my hand at the didgeridoo during a show in front of a big crowd. It was a bit daunting, but I managed to get some sound to come out the end. There was a miniature train that went around the whole grounds and made it easier to see everything. The driver let Sam feel the engine because he has a love of trains. The only complaint we had was the ibis during lunch… they wanted our food more than we did.

It was time to get wet! We headed on over to WhiteWater World, which is next to Dreamworld. This place makes adults feel like kids again and I think I had more fun than the boys. Lisa and I took it in turns going on the rides with Sam, because Mitchell was still too young and small to go on anything extreme. We stayed with him at Wiggle Bay and he had an absolute blast. Luckily it wasn't the peak season, otherwise the queues would have gone on forever. The time seemed to fly and I only wished the park stayed open later. We ended up going back to WhiteWater World a few days later because we had a SuperPass for multiple visits and I couldn't resist.

The next day we continued with the water theme at Sea World. This was going to be an extra special day because we had prearranged a dolphin encounter for Sam. We changed into our bathers and made our way over to Dolphin Cove where we were introduced to one of the instructors. Before we knew it there were two dolphins swimming up to us. One of them was to remain with us, and ironically he was named RB which is the abbreviated name for Sam's condition, retinoblastoma. Sam got to do tricks with RB, pat him and feed him slimy fish. He said the dolphin felt like a soft boiled egg to touch. This was a magical experience and another one for the memory bank. As per usual there were lots of rides, shows and fast foods.

There was no rest for the wicked and especially when I'm in charge of holidays! It was on to Warner Bros. Movie World. I only wish that Sam could have seen this place because it was very visual. Down the main street there are characters constantly coming out to meet and greet the guests. We had to explain to them and their minders that Sam was blind, and would it be OK if he could feel you to get an idea of what you 'look' like. They were very accommodating, since it's not the sort of thing that you can ask a total stranger.

Prior to us leaving home, Lisa had made contact with Guest Services to find out if there was anything they could recommend for a child with a vision impairment at the Park. As has been our experience in the past, people will go out of their way to create a special experience. Little did we know how special that would be.

We were asked to wait in the foyer of Guest Services for a one on one with none other than Bugs Bunny and Sylvester. They were amazing with the children and spent so much time with them making them laugh and playing silly games. I will never forget that moment and so grateful that I captured it on video. And this was all in silence because the characters don't talk.

While out and about in the Movieworld streets, we came across Austin Powers. We explained to him that Sam could not see and asked if Sam could feel his costume. Not only was that OK with Austin Powers, but he explained different parts of his costume to Sam and ended up having an amazing chat to him. He was absolutely wonderful. Later in the day we lined the side of the streets for the parade that routinely goes down the main street. Suddenly Lisa heard something over the loud speakers and called to me. Austin Powers was in the parade and asking "Is my friend Sam here, who I met earlier?" Thinking she must have heard incorrectly, Lisa took Sam towards the front of the crowd along the street. Austin Powers came over and seemed excited to see Sam. He asked Lisa if he could take Sam into the parade. Sam was whisked away, and before we knew it, part of the parade. He was dancing along with all the characters, walking alongside the Batmobile, and just having an awesome time. He was treated like a little prince, and loving every minute of it. Thank you Austin Powers... Groovy Baby!

In between the shows we went on all the rides and by the end of the day met all of the Warner Bros. and Looney Tunes characters. Another action-packed day for the family and a good night's sleep for four very tired individuals.

It was nearing the end of our stay and time to crank it down a gear. We decided to spend a day in Surfers Paradise and came across this funny looking vehicle called the Aquaduck, which is a land and water cruiser. It starts the tour on land and goes around to all the tourist destinations. It then makes its way onto the Broadwater, passing all the million dollar homes and a few resorts to show you how the other half live. The kids were then given an opportunity to drive the Aquaduck. Sam pushed the boundaries as usual and hit the horn, which is a big no-no on the water. However, we made it back in one piece.

While we were away Mitchell celebrated his fourth birthday, which fell on the day before Easter that year. When we arrived at the airport to go home there was an Easter Bunny walking around with an Alice in Wonderland, handing out Easter eggs to the children. It was a good way to finish off an amazing family holiday. I think Lisa was just happy to be home to have a holiday from the holiday.

Sometime after we returned home, we were invited back to the Rotary Club to share our family adventure. Sam and Lisa got up and spoke, bringing the whole trip to life, while I displayed the photos and videos which captured all of the precious moments. We have been very blessed by the people who have come into our lives.

CHAPTER 12

MY LIFE AS A BLIND BOY

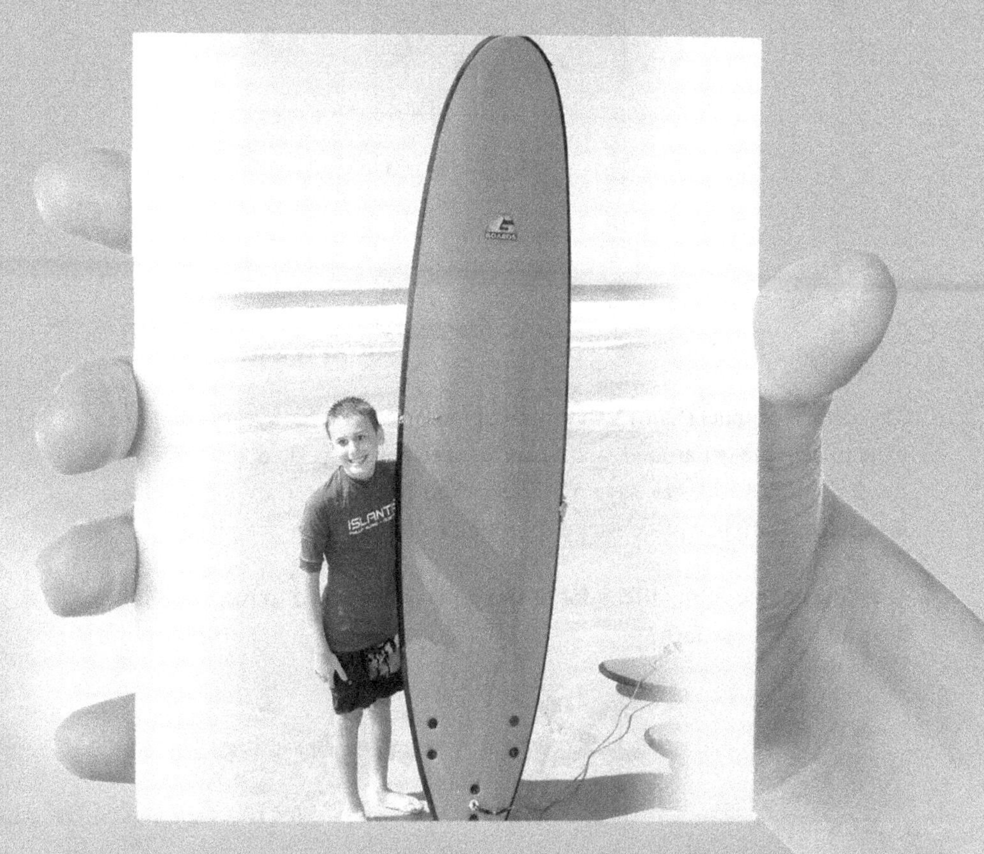

Chapter 12

My Life as A Blind Boy

(Sam)

Just because a man lacks the use of his eyes doesn't mean he lacks vision.

Stevie Wonder

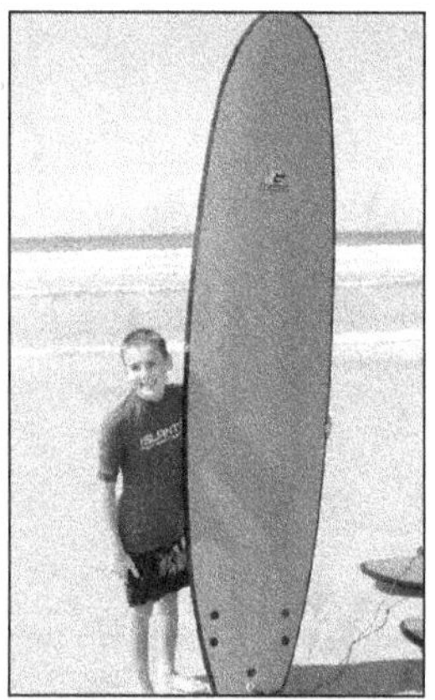

My name is Samuel (Sam) Valavanis and I am 13-and-a-half years old. I use a cane to help me get around, and I may want to have a guide dog when I grow up. I would also like to have a bionic eye to help me get around to places, especially if I'm in a place where dogs aren't allowed, such as a plane.

Over the course of my life, a lot of things have happened to me. Here is the story of my life, so far…

When I was only twelve weeks old, I was diagnosed with bilateral retinoblastoma, a rare childhood cancer of the eyes. Then began the massive treatment I was given by doctors at the Royal Children's Hospital. I don't remember much about the treatment I went through, as I was only a tiny baby then.

I was also given treatment at the Peter MacCallum Cancer Institute and the Royal Victorian Eye & Ear Hospital.

When I was three, I had my left eye surgically removed. I had started chemotherapy after I was diagnosed, as well as having cryotherapy, radiotherapy, laser therapy and multiple general anaesthetics, but the doctors were unable to cure my cancer with it, so the only option was to have my left eye removed. I don't remember much about that experience either, or how it felt at that point in time.

In 2007, at four-and-a-half-years-old, my right eye was also surgically removed as a result of the doctors not being able to treat the tumours within it, as well as the fact that it was getting dangerously close to the optic nerve, which could be really dangerous for my brain. I remember almost all of the events that occurred on that day, including the time before my surgery. Some of those events included all of my family (including my uncle, aunty and baby cousin, and both sets of grandparents) being there to support me before my surgery, as well as going down to the Starlight Express Room and dancing with my papa and saying hello to Captain Starlight.

After my operation, I took a while to adjust to living with a disability, but eventually I adapted to it. I had to learn how to navigate around my house and around my kindergarten in Patterson Lakes, where we lived at that time. But luckily I had some very helpful people on my side helping me adjust to life without sight, including my mum and dad, as well as an Early Childhood Educator, Judy Reese (who had been working with me since I was a baby), and also the teachers at my kindergarten.

In 2008, when I was six, I started in Prep at The Vision Australia School for the Blind in Burwood. Eventually I settled in, as I was surrounded by people just like me – some totally blind, some with vision in only one eye, but all were children with a vision impairment. I learnt to read and write braille (quite quickly, as I'd been learning it a little since kindergarten), although it took a while to learn contracted braille, which is a shortened form of words using certain symbols to indicate two or more letters in that one symbol. I found learning braille rather interesting and fun.

I made lots of friends at the school, some of whom I still see at a program that I go to at the Statewide Vision Resource Centre (SVRC) called Support Skills, for children in Grades Four to Ten. Some of the activities at Support Skills include cooking, PE, maths, learning about technology, art, music and daily living skills.

The following year, my parents enrolled me at Berwick Chase Primary School, where I was the only student with a disability there at the time. By then I was in Grade One. I was a bit nervous being the only blind student at my school, but eventually I adapted to it and really enjoyed going there. The school helped my transition become a lot easier by buying special equipment for me (including a Perkins Brailler, a talking calculator and a Mountbatten Brailler), as well as having a specialist aid to help me with mobility skills, and also having a Teacher's Aid to help me in the classroom.

A year after I started at Berwick Chase, Vision Australia sold the land of the Vision Australia School, as they were going to build a housing estate on that land, and from then on I went to Berwick Chase full time. I took away lots of memories from Vision Australia, and from then on I learnt braille individually, assisted by a Visiting Teacher, Melissa Bowyer, from SVRC. I also now had a full-time Orientation & Mobility (O&M) teacher, Gail Stinchcombe, who worked at Vision Australia's head office in Kooyong.

In 2015, I started Year Seven at Timbarra College, a P-9 (Prep to Year Nine) school in Berwick. I was really excited to start secondary school.

Also towards the end of 2015, I found out that Melissa would not continue as my Visiting Teacher in 2016 (as she had been my visiting teacher since 2010), and that she would be replaced by Sue Matthews, a Visiting Teacher whom I also knew from Vision Australia where I went to school in 2008 and 2009. Sue has worked with me ever since the start of 2016, currently visiting my school twice a week, as did Melissa.

I have also had a lot of special experiences in my life. Some of them may stand out more than others. For example, going to Disneyland and the Gold Coast really stood out for me because they were really fun things to have done with my family.

In 2006, I was lucky enough to be made an Honorary Junior Firefighter at the Eastern Hill Fire Station in East Melbourne. I did lots of fun things on that day, including dressing up as a fireman, using a fire hose, riding through the city in a fire engine, going up in a cherry picker, eating lunch with the firefighters and receiving a teddy bear that I named Terry at the very beginning of the day. My dad also made a special 'Fireman Sam' T-shirt for me to wear on the day, since I really loved Fireman Sam at the time.

In 2007, I went on a day trip from Moorabbin Airport to the Werribee Police and Fire Stations and then on to Williamstown with the State Emergency Services (SES) and Coast Guard. All the major Victorian organisations were involved, including Victoria Police, CFA, SES and Coast Guard. The event was shown on the *National Nine News* that evening.

In the same year, just before I lost my sight completely, *The Today Show* announced that my parents had won a 'Week of Wishes' competition that they had been entered in by our neighbours for a trip to Disneyland. I was really happy at Disneyland, and it had been my first time flying on an aeroplane, so there were a lot of new experiences for me. In the USA, we stayed at the Paradise Pier hotel in Anaheim and the Crowne Plaza hotel in Beverly Hills, since we also stayed there for a few nights.

I was also lucky enough to be given a tour by QANTAS of a Boeing 747 prior to the trip. I got to look at the cockpit and also first class.

In 2007 and 2010, my parents organised and held two Family Fun Days to raise money for Beyond Sight, which is an auxiliary of the RCH, and to raise awareness for children with retinoblastoma and also to raise enough money to pay for much-needed equipment required by RCH doctors in the Ophthalmology Department.

In 2010, the Noble Park Rotary offered to send my family on a trip to the Gold Coast in Queensland. I really had fun up there, and I really enjoyed all the theme parks that we went to. The parks we went to were Movieworld, Seaworld, Dreamworld and WhiteWater World, and some of the rides we went on were The Tower of Terror, The Cyclone, The Green Room, The Bermuda Triangle and The Flume.

In 2012, my parents announced that we were going by car up to Sydney for a week. We did lots of fun things in Sydney, including going on the Monorail, going up the Sydney Tower Eye, visiting the Sydney Opera House, the Royal Botanic Gardens, the Rocks and the Sydney Harbour Bridge.

Some other holidays and destinations we've been to as a family include camping trips to such places as Lakes Entrance, Ballarat, Warrnambool, Swan Hill, Mount Gambier, Victor Harbour, Bendigo, Mildura and Renmark, just to name a few. More recent camping trips have been taken in our exciting new caravan.

In October 2014, my family and I went to the Channel 9 studios in Melbourne to see 'Kids WB' being filmed. We met Lauren Phillips and Shane Crawford, the show's hosts, as well as Jo Hall and Livinia Nixon around the studios.

I've also met some other famous people including Andy Griffiths (children's author), Stig Wemyss (actor, producer and narrator), Jules Lund (TV and radio personality), Louise Baxter (CEO of the Starlight Children's Foundation) and Tony Jones (Channel 9 news and sports reporter).

In June 2015, my family were invited to attend Vision Australia's tenth Anniversary Cocktail Party in the city, and Mum and I were asked to speak about how Vision Australia has helped us over the years. We met some special people there, including April Wilkinson, Vision Australia's Relations Officer; Ron Hooton, the CEO of Vision Australia; David Hall, the CEO of Jetstar; and David Mann, who works at the 3AW studios in the city. After Mum and I presented our speeches, these people were so impressed that they offered us a number of amazing opportunities: free passes to the annual Carols by Candlelight (as well as speaking again in front of 150 VIP's there), a free trip to anywhere in Australia, and a tour of the 3AW studios in the city.

In July 2015, Dad and I participated in Run Melbourne, with the famous Australian Paralympian Jessica "Jess" Gallagher, as well as another family with two girls who had a vision-impaired sister. I had also appeared in several media promotions in the month before the run, including Vision Australia Radio, dressing in a Superman costume to promote the event. Jess and I did an interview on the Vision Australia Radio show *Behind the Scenes*, presented by John Sheridan. We also took part in a photoshoot and the photos were then featured in newspapers and posted online.

As already mentioned, David Mann from 3AW had given us the opportunity to have a tour of the 3AW studios in the city, and we went in to have a look around on July 3, 2015. David met us in the lobby, and gave Dad and I security passes to access all areas of the studio, including areas that the general public would not usually be able to access. We met Jason, one of the security guards there, and proceeded up to the seventh floor, where the studios were. On arrival I met people such as Bruce Mansfield, Jordan Tunbridge, Leigh Matthews (Hawthorn football legend and former coach of several clubs) and Tony Tardio, just to name a few. When I got to one of the rooms in the studio, I found a stuffed dodo bird sitting on the mixing desk waiting for me, which I got to take home. I also spoke to fellow radio stations in Sydney and Perth with Tony over the communication system. I even got to go into the neighbouring radio studio, Magic 1278, which had closed up for the night, as it was 7:30 pm by that time (we got there just before 7 pm). I found out that the music at night is programmed by a computer during the day. After a good look around, it was time to go, so we went back down to the lobby and Dad gave his security pass back to Jason, who said I could keep mine as a souvenir of the trip, which I greatly appreciated. We thanked them very much for everything, and then went home.

Also around that time, I was lucky enough to be invited to the Bolinda Audio recording studios in Tullamarine, where Stig Wemyss records audiobooks for people to listen to. When we went in, Stig took us to the recording booth where he records the books, and I got the chance to interview him and pretend I was the host of my own TV show, as well as record my own narrative. After that, we looked around the warehouse at the back of the building, where they store all the audiobooks and distribute them out to shops and libraries all around the country. I met Joe, the man in the warehouse who helps distribute the books and I also got to meet the staff who work in the office, except the boss Rebecca, who was away on business in Queensland. The team at Bolinda kindly gave me a lot of audiobooks to take home with me and listen to. We thanked everyone very much for their time and went home.

In September we went on a holiday to Perth, thanks to David and the team from Jetstar, and did lots of amazing things there. We went to a theme park called Adventure World, Rottnest Island by ferry, Fremantle, Cottesloe, Scarborough, Hillarys Boat Harbour, Lake Joondalup, Bunbury, Margaret River and much more. We had organised to meet a blind girl named Ally and her family at the Kings Park and Botanic Garden, and had a picnic there. I also met some of my mum's family I had never met before. We took lots of photos and bought lots of memorabilia to take home with us. It was a very fun trip.

In December, on Christmas Eve, we attended Carols by Candlelight at the Sidney Myer Music Bowl in the city. We were also invited by April Wilkinson, whom we saw at the cocktail party, to attend the VIP party before the Carols started. Mum and I were again asked to speak in front of the 150 guests and dignitaries at the event, with Ron Hooton introducing us. Everyone was very impressed with our speeches, and we were congratulated by many people afterwards, including 3AW radio presenter Denis Walter and his wife. We enjoyed the carols very much, and were very tired by the time we got home. It was a night to remember.

I've also had a lot of fun experiences with Camp Quality, Challenge and the Starlight Children's Foundation. I've been on many camps with them, including family camps and camps for kids. I've made lots of friends with the other kids and staff who are a part of these organisations and camps.

Overall, a lot of things have happened to me in my life, including some things I never would have expected. For example, I never would have thought that I would meet and make friends with some really famous Australian celebrities.

Some special achievements in my life include being named Science Captain at Berwick Chase Primary School in Grade Six and being named one of the Starlight Ambassadors for the Starlight 25-year anniversary celebrations.

I've also tried a number of sports too. Some of these include blind cricket, goalball and swimming. However, out of those three sports, I found goalball was the sport I really want to play the most. But if you play in any one of those three sports, you have a chance of being able to represent Australia internationally if you become good.

I learnt to play the piano, using the Suzuki Method. Dad would drive me for an hour to an 8 am Saturday morning lesson, learning from a piano teacher named Daphne Proietto. I even got to play in a number of concerts with her other students. She was a great teacher, but I chose to give it up. However, I am now learning the keyboard at Timbarra, my high school.

Since I can play the piano well, whenever I hear a song I like on the radio or the TV, I can play it on the piano off by heart because I find it is such fun doing this. I am also really good at harmonising songs on the piano or keyboard.

It feels so good whenever I try something new. I love trying new and different foods. Mum says she cannot fill me up.

A great passion I have is my love of rollercoasters and thrill rides. My dad calls me an "adrenalin junkie". For example, when my family and I went to the Gold Coast, I went on pretty much all the rides, even the scary ones, for children my age and height, and this was a lot of fun. So it wouldn't surprise you that when I wanted to go on the Sea Viper at Seaworld, and I was too short for the ride, I burst into tears, for I was only seven years old then. However, next time we go to the Gold Coast, I'm confident I'll be able to go on this ride, because I've grown a lot since then, and I should be hitting my growth spurt soon.

A great skill I have is mapping out new areas, even if I've only been there a few times. I am proud of this skill because when I started school, I didn't know where anything was, and now I know my school like the back of my hand. And now that I've been at secondary school for a while, I've mapped out a lot of the area quite confidently, and I also have lots of friends to help me find my way.

Some of my favourite subjects are Geography and History. I really find these subjects interesting and fun to learn. One day, I hope to travel the world, and use my amazing Geography and History knowledge to amaze and surprise others.

As well as Geography and History, I also love learning about general knowledge. For example, what was the first spacecraft to land on the Moon, about the Empire State Building, and much more. I always want to learn more about the world and some of the amazing people and things in it.

Some amazing abilities I have are being able to use echolocation, as well as my remarkable hearing. I use echolocation to help me find where I am in a room or to find a certain object, either by clapping my hands or clicking my tongue. Because I have no sight my hearing is quite sensitive, and it allows me to hear things up to at least 5–10 metres away, including things that other people can't hear. I think this will be an important ability to have in the future because if there was a burglary in the next street I would be able to hear it and call the police!

When I'm older, I want to study Medicine, because I really want to be an Anaesthetist. Some of the first places I want to work are the Royal Children's Hospital, Royal Victorian Eye & Ear Hospital and Peter MacCallum Cancer Institute, because they all did their best to help me when I had cancer. But firstly I want to work at the RCH because they're the ones who removed the tumours from both of my eyes, and I would like to give something back to them in return.

In the future, I hope to achieve a lot of things, including travelling all around the world, going back to Disneyland and the Gold Coast and appearing on TV for the first time in a while, as I have been on television on various occasions and loved it. Maybe I could appear as a news reporter, because I'd really like to read the news one day.

If you put your mind to it, in the end you can do anything. It doesn't matter whether you have a disability or impairment, or if you feel like you can't do anything. What matters most is that you do what you've always wanted to do and, more importantly, have lots of fun doing it!

Mim's Poem for Sam

Written for: Samuel (Sam) Valavanis
By: Meredith (Mim) Boxall
30th August 2007

Who Is This Boy?

Who is this little boy of five that's forever on my mind?
Who's locked deep within my heart, one of a 'Special Kind'.
Who loves to sing and dance and play, who's just like me and you.
In fact, there's nothing in this world this little boy can't do.
He sprawls out upon the floor amusing himself with toys,
And when he's finished, up he pops to play with the girls and boys.
He'll sit with me upon my knee and say "Let's go to Mars".
And next I know we're on the mat amongst buses, trains and cars.
When is it morning tea time? What's for lunch today?
What time will Mummy pick me up? About 4:30 I say.
He has his loveable 'Ol' Pooh Bear' that went with him to Disneyland.
Where ever he goes 'Pooh' goes, he's always in his hand.
Ask him about his Elephant known to all as 'Heidi-Ho'.
Ask him any question and he is sure to know.
What colour is a fire engine, RED he shouts with glee.
And who's just been to Disneyland? Oh Mum, Dad, Mitch and me.
So, who is this little boy you ask, the one of a 'Special Kind'?
His name is SAMUEL VALAVANIS and he is totally blind.
He has an adoring family who are always there for him.
His baby brother Mitchell, Mother Lisa and Father Jim.
And who am I who knows this boy who's forever on my mind.
My name is Mim, at crèche I take care of him, and he sure is of a 'Special Kind'!

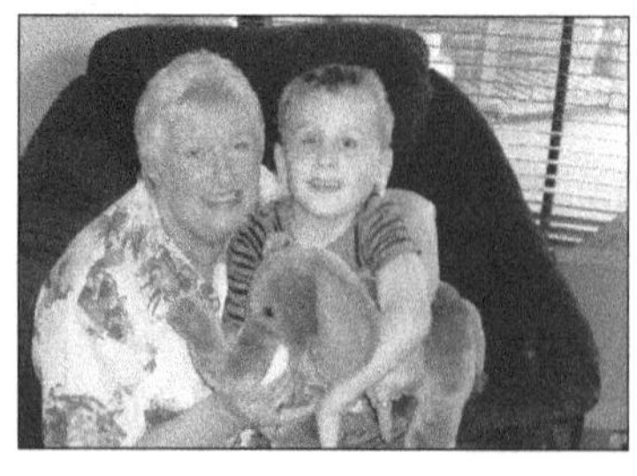

CHAPTER 13

'SAM-ECDOTES'
(SAM'S ANECDOTES)

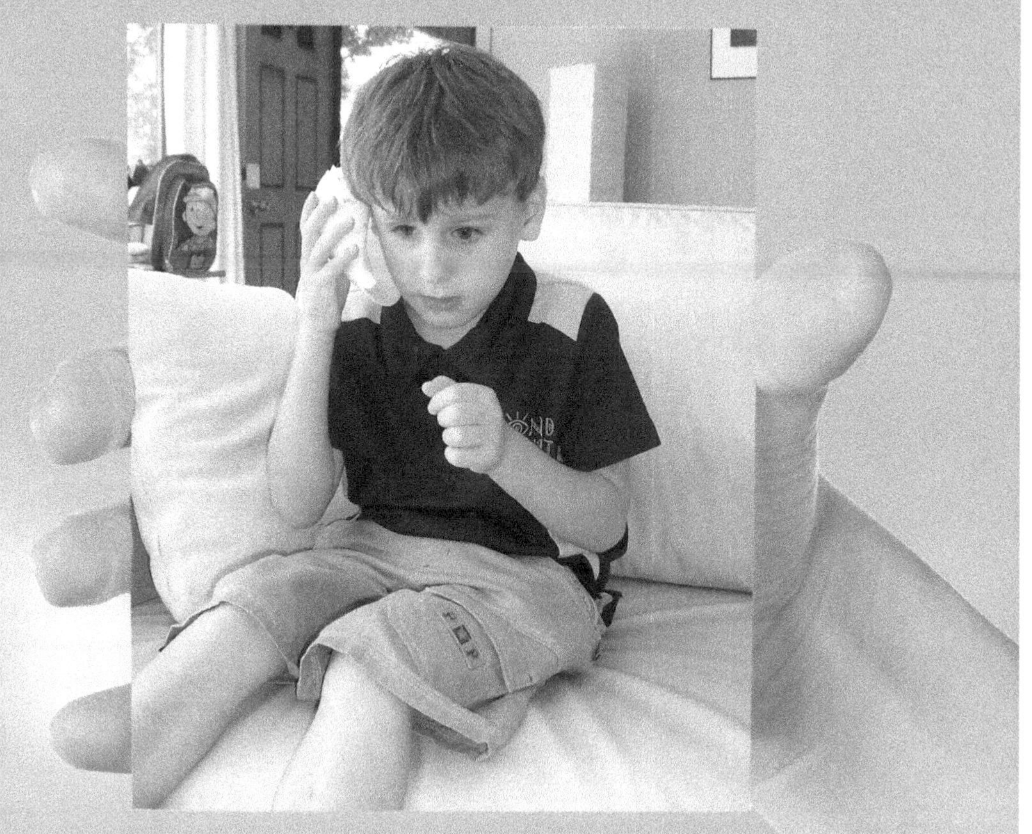

Chapter 13

'Sam-Ecdotes'
(Sam's Anecdotes)

(Lisa)

Our fate lies within us.
You only have to be brave enough to see it

Merida – 'Brave'
Walt Disney Pictures
Pixar Animation Studios

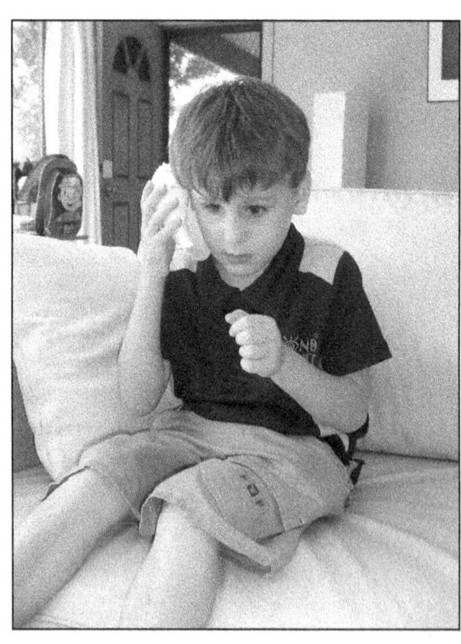

Despite what Sam and our family have been through, there have been a lot of laughs over the years. Whether there have been funny things that have happened, silly things that Sam has said, or stupid situations Sam has gotten into, we have tried to put a positive light-hearted spin on the hand that fate has dealt us all. Some people may look at me a bit strangely with the things that we do or say, but I always say that it's either laugh or cry about what's happened. Being sad or crying about it is not going to fix the problem or change what has happened, so we may as well look at things in a positive way, have a laugh and not take life so seriously.

Below I have put together some of these little bits and pieces. Just a list, in no particular order, that have come to mind. Hope you have as much of a giggle as we have had along the way…

Sam was looking for something in his room one day and couldn't seem to find it. I was listening to him from the next room. Then I heard the click of the light switch to turn it on. "That's better," says Sam. Putting the light on makes such a difference when you are blind!

Sam comes into my room and sits on the bed. He put his hand on the bed. "I see you have a new doona cover Mum, it looks great."

When I will get ready to go out somewhere special, he will give me a hug before I leave and say "You look beautiful Mum".

There have been occasions where I have accidentally (honestly!) walked Sam into walls, poles, tripped up or down steps. I'll always say, "Sorry Sam, I forgot you were blind". "Oh Mum!" I get from him.

Sam will be running around the house like a maniac with his brother and sister, then slam into a door or wall. "Stupid wall, why did the builders put it there?" Always somebody else's fault.

In Grade Two at school Sam's class were discussing being blind and guide dogs. Somebody asked Sam if he would get a guide dog when he is an adult. His response was "I might get a guide dog… or I might just get a wife!"

When Sam was designated a 'House' at school, he was put into red house. He was very unhappy, as his favourite colour was blue. The first time he had to wear his house colour of red, I said "Don't worry, your T-shirt is blue". A little white/blue lie helps calm an upset child.

Sam was running around like a crazy boy at school at pick up time with his younger brother – they were chasing each other around the bright red metal fire hose reel box. Sam slammed into the corner of it and split his head open. He started to scream, "It happened because I'm blind". To which I replied "No, it happened because you were being silly and not listening to me when I said not to do it". He soon shut up.

Jim has nicknamed Sam's cane 'Michael', 'aka Michael Caine'.

With Sam being blind, it does have some advantages. I have been known to send him out the door in the morning with two different socks on, as I couldn't find a matching pair. If they feel the same, that's ok for Sam.

Sam ended up in an arm half-cast last year. When I was at karate with Mitchell, I received a phone call from Jim, asking if I felt like a trip to the emergency room when I got home. After getting home, I found out that Sam had jumped off the top of his loft bed and onto the floor. When I asked why he did it, his response was "Mitchell does it". He realised that the only downside of his plan was that Mitchell can also see where he is landing.

Those who know us personally will know that our home is a little 'tidily challenged'. Yet, if I have lost something, Sam will quite often be the one to be able to find it. Eyes aren't always an advantage.

Sam will quite often catch me out. My weakness is chocolate. I don't care how much a Mum loves her kids, but sometimes there is no sharing. I can hide away from sight and fuel my addiction. But then Sam will come into the room to talk to me. "You've been eating chocolate Mum, I can smell it on your breath." Damn it, caught out.

Sam is an absolutely crazy daredevil. He has no sense of fear. When it comes to theme park rides, they cannot be big enough, fast enough or wild enough for Sam. He will take me on a scary ride, which I do love, but will freak out and have a spontaneous 'Tourette's' outburst. We will get off the ride and Sam will be in fits of laughter at me and all of the other screamers on the ride. "You were so scared" he will say. It's alright for him, he can't see the point on a ride where you fear it will slam into the ground and kill you.

At Halloween last year, it was decided that instead of terrifying people out on the street with 'Trick or Treating', we would stay at home and greet people who came knocking at our door. Sam wanted to meet kids at the door looking like a zombie, with his prosthetic eyes out, holding them out at people and stating "I have my eyes on you". We decided against this, thinking it would just scare people a little bit too much. Some things are even too realistically scary for Halloween.

At kid's parties, Sam was an absolute champ at 'Pin the Tail on the Donkey'. He always had an upper hand on the other kids when they were blindfolded. It was nothing new for him.

When Sam first became totally blind, he was quite angry and sad about it. "Why can't the doctors make me see again?" Then he started changing the way he would look at the situation. "I hate being blind. But if I wasn't blind, I couldn't do braille and I really like doing braille".

When I was working two days a week after having Mitchell, my Mum and Dad would look after him. Sam was going to the Vision Australia School then, and my Dad would pick him up from the taxi drop-off point and take him back to their house. After work, I would pick both boys up from my parents' house. One day I came to pick them up and asked what the boys had been up to. "We don't know if we should tell you" my Mum said. After giving them a suspicious look, Mum told me that both boys had climbed up on to the shed roof. A blind five-year-old and his two-year-old brother. No, having no sight had definitely not slowed Sam down.

CHAPTER 14

LIFE LESSONS
WHAT HAVE WE LEARNED…

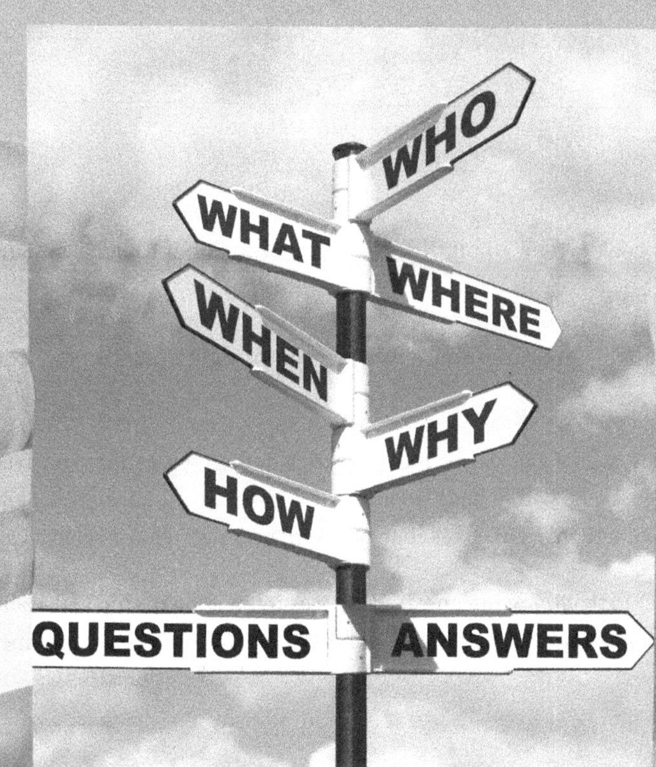

Chapter 14

Life Lessons – What Have We Learned...

(Jim and Lisa)

Change your thoughts and
you change your world.

Norman Vincent Peale

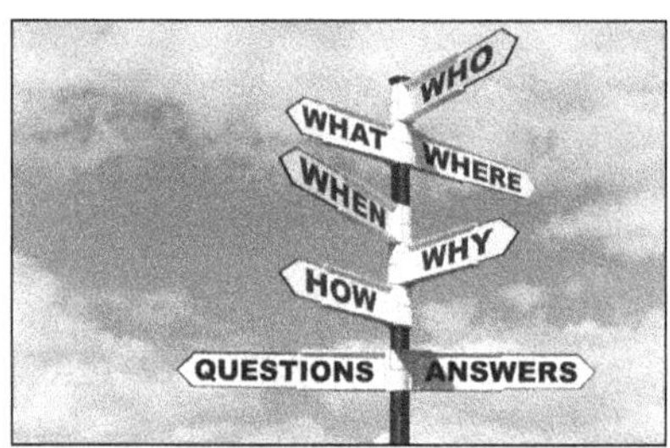

In writing this book together, both Jim and I have been through a huge amount of, well, 'stuff'.

It has made us relive our time since Sam was born, right up until now, as a blind teenager.

The process has brought up all of the memories and emotions that we lived through, both good and bad. It has also made us realise that we have grown and learnt a lot about not only ourselves, but each other throughout this journey.

We each answered the following questions. It was interesting to stop and really think about our answers. Some were so obvious, but some even surprised me.

Jim

What are you grateful for?

- The fact that we still have Sam in our lives
- The fact that he has adapted amazingly well to life with a vision impairment and thriving
- This experience has changed us as people for the better
- We look at life very differently now and have reprioritised what's important to us
- We have learnt to appreciate the little things
- It took me a long time to switch my way of thinking because I was in the mindset of the things that we couldn't do with Sam rather than being grateful for the things we could do with him

What have you learnt about yourself?

- That I'm a lot more resilient than I thought I was
- I place more importance on family now than anything else
- I appreciate the little things and don't worry about things I can't control anymore
- We have learnt to live life to the fullest and make the most of every experience
- I want to help others by sharing our experience and story
- I love meeting new people and getting to know them on a deep level, not just the superficial small talk

- You need to stop and 'smell the roses' by being and living in the moment

- I've learnt that my wife is the 'rock' in our family and that I couldn't have done it without her

What have you learnt about other people?

- Strangers will go out of their way to help you in any way they can

- You learn who your true friends are

- A lot of people have a genuine interest in our story

- There are a lot of good people out there who do great things that goes unnoticed and unappreciated

- People open up to you more easily once they see your vulnerable side

- "There's many ways to skin a cat!" There's more than one solution to a problem if you know where to look or who to speak to

What would you have done differently now that you know what you know?

- Speak to more people about natural remedies and alternative therapies

- Seriously think about whether to bombard Sam with so many chemicals when he was so young, now knowing the eventual outcome

- Join a parent support group

- Get involved with the charities a lot earlier than what we did. We waited till Sam was in remission until we got involved (i.e. Starlight, Camp Quality, Challenge)

- Seek assistance from allied health professionals much earlier

- Open up to friends and family you feel you can confide in
- Join a club or sports group to socialise and help with your healing
- Exercise and stay active to reduce stress, anxiety, insomnia, depression
- Eat well and use supplements (not medication)

What are your daily rituals or things you do habitually to keep you sane and grounded?

- Take time out for myself. May be going for a walk, ride, reading a book, bath, massage, movie, listen to music, audiobook
- Talk to my wife Lisa about what's on my mind (better out than in!)
- Watch what goes into my body (nutrition and supplements)
- Keep moving every day and get the heart pumping. Don't be sedentary
- Have family time but also look after yourself and your sanity. Quiet time where you can inwardly reflect and reenergise
- Reduce the negativity in your life (peer groups, social media, family members, media, toxins, chemicals)

What would you like people to get out of sharing our experience?

- Inspire people to never give up no matter what challenges or adversities you are faced with in life
- Give people a sense of hope that there is light at the end of the tunnel, even though you can't see it at the time

- Whether you have a disability or not you can live a long, happy and fulfilled life
- Don't place limitations on yourself and be told how to live your life. Live it on your terms and be the master of your own destiny
- Learn to appreciate the little things and be grateful for what you have
- Don't wait for tomorrow to make a bucket list/goals/plans... do it today and start ticking them off one by one before it's too late and keep adding to it as you go

Lisa

What am I grateful for?

- Breathing, simply being alive
- Sam still being with us
- Family and friends
- My health and that of my family

What have I learnt about myself?

- I am a lot stronger than I ever thought I was
- I have learnt to trust my gut/motherly instincts
- I am not to blame for what happened to Sam
- We are not 'victims'
- I am learning what I want to do 'when I grow up'

What have I learnt about others?

- A lot of people's ideas and opinions relate to their own issues and have nothing to do with me
- Everybody processes and deals with things (stress, grief, etc.) differently
- We found out that many people we thought of as 'friends' really were not there for us in our time of need
- On the other hand, other people who we thought of as only acquaintances really stepped up to become absolute life-savers for us
- I've learnt to spot the people whose life values are very different to ours
- I realise that there are many negative people in the world
- We are learning that it is to our family's benefit to remove people with 'toxic' attitudes from our lives

What would I have done differently now that I know what I know?

- Trust my own judgement
- Be more in control of my family's issues and wellbeing
- Don't self-blame
- Not to have negative thoughts and behaviours – they don't fix the problem, but simply just put you in a dark place
- Try to look for a positive in every situation
- Been more aware and knowledgeable about Sam's treatment options, side effects and long term consequences. Also know more about alternative and supplementary treatments

What are your daily rituals or things you do habitually to keep you sane and grounded?

- No idea, hence the reason I am insane!
- Breathe. A wonderful friend kept reminding me of that on my wedding day
- Tea. Keep calm and put the kettle on. Having a quiet cuppa in a fancy-pants cup and saucer puts me in a calmer mood
- Ideally:
  - Meditation
  - Eating well and looking after myself
  - Exercise
  - Think about what I'm grateful for in life

What would you like people to get out of sharing our experience?

- To not feel that they are alone in their journey or grief
- There is a light at the end of the tunnel, no matter how long the tunnel seems
- Try to look for a positive in every negative
- Trust your instincts or inner voice
- Don't be afraid to question doctors, they can get it wrong sometimes
- Ask questions, no matter how stupid you think it is
- Have the courage to speak up
- Be knowledgeable about all your treatment options
- Leave guilt behind. It is a very useless and toxic emotion

CHAPTER 15

LIVE LIFE TO THE FULLEST

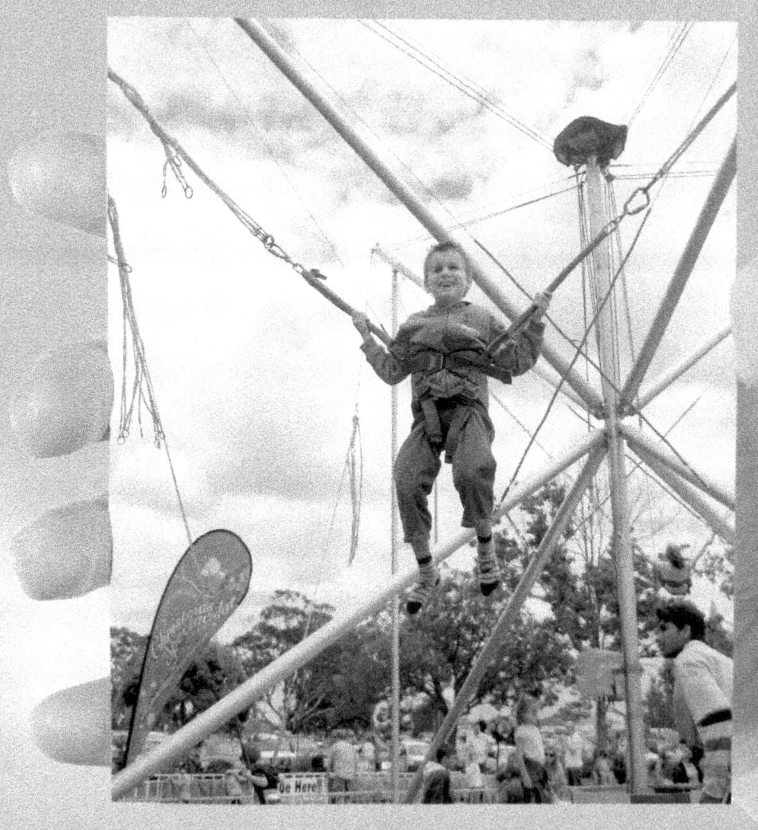

Chapter 15

Live Life to The Fullest

(Jim)

> *Don't be a spectator on the sidelines.*
> *You need to step into the game of life!*
>
> **Unknown**

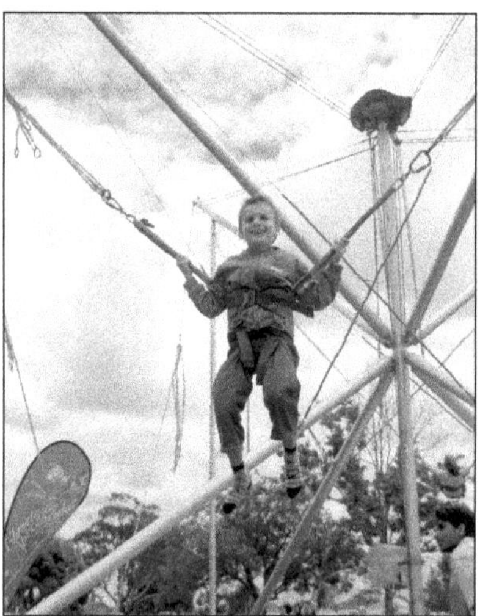

What is the meaning of life? That is the 64,000-dollar question! Why are we here and what is our purpose for existing?

When you go through such a traumatic event, whether it be yourself or a loved one, you look at the world very differently and truly understand how fragile life can be. It's the little things that you learn to appreciate and you thank your lucky stars that the sun will rise tomorrow to bring a new day. We kept saying to ourselves that no matter how bad our situation was, there is always someone else that is worse off than you.

As difficult as it may be to comprehend at the time, you have to accept your circumstances and look at the bigger picture. Appreciate what you DO have, not what you DON'T have. Yes, our twelve-week-old was diagnosed with a rare eye cancer and he had a visual impairment, but the main thing was that we still had him. We remained positive and focused on getting him better and nothing else mattered. We had tunnel vision on his health and wellbeing!

The treatment was tough on the whole family and took a lot of time and energy, but the end goal was to save our son's life. It was a means to an end and I would've run through a brick wall if it would have helped Sam.

We were extremely fortunate to have tremendous support from family and friends. I believe this helped us enormously to keep it all together. A positive attitude and outlook is paramount to helping the person going through the treatment, to draw strength from others. They feel reassured and energised by those around them, as opposed to someone that is constantly surrounded by doom and gloom, along with negative energy. It is hard enough as it is, let alone being dragged down when your immune system has been compromised.

In my opinion, being rich and wealthy shouldn't equate to having material THINGS and possessions. True wealth is all about life experiences, culture, surrounding yourself with good family and friends that support you and bring out the best in you.

Life is so precious and can be taken from us in the blink of an eye, so we should all have goals or a 'bucket list', but that bucket should be empty when we come to the end of our time here on earth.

Through this disease, as horrible as it is, we have met some wonderful people and had some amazing experiences. The generosity of some people, organisations and charities still ceases to amaze me.

It has allowed us to push the boundaries of what we initially thought for life with a vision impaired child and live outside our comfort zone. It has given us the opportunity to do things that we normally wouldn't think of doing and at the same time given Sam the confidence to be more independent and curious to give anything a go. His zest for life certainly keeps us going and also gives us a sense of hope for his future.

Sam has a lot of fight and spirit in him and is an inspiration to all of those who come into contact with him. He has no fear in him and because of the fact that he can't see what he's about to do, will attempt things that adults would think twice about doing or refuse to do altogether!

Whether it be surfing, snow skiing, riding a rollercoaster or a treetop high ropes course, Sam jumps at the opportunity with an open mind and a free spirit to experience all that life has to offer. His sense of adventure has rubbed off on the whole family and we have recently purchased a caravan to explore every 'nook and cranny' of this great land that we call home.

For your health and wellbeing, it is important to take some time out for yourself each and every day, doing something as simple as going for a walk or whatever else you feel compelled to do, (i.e. run, meditate, yoga, Pilates, Tai Chi, exercise, ride, swim). It helps clear your mind, collect all your thoughts and relieve tension for the day… it also gets the blood pumping and your muscles moving. It just makes you feel alive. It is important to make this a habit, so whether you choose to do it alone or with somebody else, that doesn't matter... JUST DO IT!!!

Turn off all of your electronic devices; your iPad, your smart phone, TV, radio and all of the other distractions we surround ourselves with and talk one-on-one with somebody at a deep level. Make a connection with them and really pay attention to each and every word they're saying, without thinking about what you're going to say next. Learn to be a good listener and take it all in, empathise with the other person and put yourself in their shoes. How are they feeling? How can you make their day better by how you respond? Talk about them and their life first before you talk about yourself. We all do this without thinking subconsciously, but make yourself aware and after a while it will come naturally.

Make a bucket list. Be a kid again. Remember when we were kids, we used to dream, "I wanna be this and I wanna do that". It is something to look forward to and gives you an appreciation of life and a sense of achievement, not to mention an unforgettable experience. When we grow up we let life get in the way and we stop dreaming. We should never forget where we came from and where we want to go.

Follow your heart and be true to yourself. We only get one chance at life so why not live it to the fullest. Treat every day like it may be your last. Live in the moment, and as the famous saying goes, "Stop and smell the roses". Cherish those little things that seem to come and go without being acknowledged. Appreciate what you have and be thankful to those around you, because life is a blessing.

What is your reason for getting up in the morning? What could you not do without in your life? Apart from coffee or chocolate! What will trigger you to make a change? Don't wait for a life-changing event to make you snap out of the 'rat race' and reprioritise what's important to you. You can do it today, or tomorrow if you want to sleep on it. It is a decision YOU and only YOU can make. You have to want it bad enough that you'll step out of your comfort zone and do whatever it takes. We all have 24 hours in a day, but it's how we choose to utilise them that's the difference. Learn to say "no" to things that aren't in your values and beliefs. Initially you may feel selfish or uncomfortable, but you need to look after number one first and then divide your time up over the other things that are important to you, (i.e. your family, friends, job, hobbies, sports etc.). We all deserve happiness and a sense of belonging, not to mention feeling loved.

Having played a number of sports for most of my childhood and well into my twenties, I always knew about the power of positive thinking and having a positive mental attitude. Just being in a positive frame of mind can make a huge difference to how you deal with obstacles in your life. Surround yourself with positive people. Negative people always look at the world with the glass half empty and want to drag others around them down to their level.

Visualise yourself doing things that make you happy. Take time out in your day to use your mind's eye and transport yourself to another place. It may seem a little 'woo woo', but this can quite quickly help you recharge your batteries and should not be underestimated.

Take up an activity or hobby which is of interest to you and makes you focus on something other than the mundane events of everyday life. This is also a good way of making new friends and associations with like-minded people who have similar interests.

Make plans for the future… three, six and twelve months down the track, which will give you something to look forward to. Plan that weekend away you keep putting off, go hot air ballooning, learn to surf, take up dancing. Do whatever you wanted to do when you were a child and kept putting off because life got in the way.

The definition of insanity is doing the same thing over and over again and expecting to get a different result (Albert Einstein). Have mental health breaks, or have a holiday every six months. Make an effort to get away from the rat race, even if it's only for a weekend. Otherwise the days turn into weeks, which then turn into months and before you know it, years have gone by and you've achieved nothing, nor experienced anything. You are merely existing and not living.

Life is a gift and each day is as precious as the next. Don't take the days for granted because once the sun sets, it's gone forever. We should be grateful and thankful for everything we have in our lives and tell those close to us how much they mean. Something as simple as a handwritten card or letter, an email or a text message, some flowers or chocolates, can have such a positive impact on them.

It's not that difficult to live a fulfilled and joyous life. Here are some things I've found which can give you the life you've always wanted and truly deserve. You don't have to do each and every one, but you might want to see what works best for you.

- Have a purpose. What is your reason for getting up in the morning?
- Do what you love and love what you do
- Have a work–life balance. Don't live to work but work to live
- Inspire others and be inspired
- Connect with others and be engaged socially with family, friends and groups
- Take time out for yourself
- Exercise and have regular movement in your life
- Have hobbies and interests
- Constantly revise your goals, make plans for the week/month/year
- Be self-motivated or find something that motivates you
- Be a student who is constantly learning. Expand your mind
- Choose your circle of influence wisely (you are the average of the five closest people in your life)
- Have plenty of rest and sleep. You shouldn't be waking up tired
- Have a mentor/s. It helps you grow, gives you direction and keeps you accountable
- Have faith in a higher power, whether it be spirituality, religion or other
- Have family getaways and holidays
- Surround yourself with positive people and choose your peer groups
- Be grateful and thankful for what you have

- Move outside your comfort zone, push the boundaries
- Give yourself new experiences
- Don't put limitations on yourself
- Have one-on-one time with your spouse/partner and each child individually
- Challenge yourself
- Don't stress about the little things. Put your energy into things that matter
- Give back – volunteer your time and/or money to charities
- Good nutrition, watch what you eat – Just Eat Real Food (JERF)
- Drink plenty of water, ideally filtered and good quality
- Cut out or reduce your intake of alcohol
- Get 15–20 minutes of sunlight each day
- Don't forget to smile and laugh
- Control the controllables
- Be the master of your destiny. Take control of your life
- Keep your attitude in check
- Be disciplined
- Have a daily ritual (It can take up to 28 days to form a habit)
- Take some time out for yourself to refresh and recharge
- Don't hold on to negative thoughts, learn to forgive and let go of resentment, jealousy, hate and anger
- Nobody is perfect, but do something each day to be the best version of yourself. Always strive to be the best you can be
- Look after yourself first and foremost so that you can be there for others

- Grow old gracefully and embrace it
- Don't be superficial
- Make the best of your situation
- Hold yourself accountable and take responsibility for your actions
- Don't settle for mediocrity
- Deal with whatever is in front of you at the time
- Be resilient, never give up
- Confide in someone
- Always have hope, inner strength and courage
- Remember that there's always someone worse off than you. We all have struggles and challenges
- Be accepting of others no matter what their ability or disability
- Love each day above ground and live in the moment
- Be mindful
- Prioritise what's important
- Stop worrying about money (it's the biggest cause of relationship breakdowns and unhealthy)
- Learn how to deal with stress. Find your release valve
- You can't be everything to everyone, so don't spread yourself thin
- Know yourself and your body
- Find a way to stay grounded and balanced - meditation, yoga, Pilates
- Trust your gut instinct
- Keep things simple and don't overcomplicate them
- Don't stress and worry about things that are out of your control

- Don't dwell on things
- Be forgiving
- Be engaged
- Be involved in your community
- Be happy but remember it's OK to feel other emotions too
- Love yourself
- Love your life
- Improve your life if you don't like things. It's up to you to make a change
- Believe in yourself
- Be passionate
- Age is a state of mind, an attitude
- Celebrate each and every birthday
- Do something nice for others
- Have a positive outlook and mindset
- Don't be a victim
- Minimise stress in your life
- If you're on prescription drugs, change your lifestyle and/or diet to get off them totally if possible (NOTE: consult your physician first)
- Stretch and stay flexible
- Keep an open mind
- Don't be the norm, be the exception
- Don't be afraid to change as a person
- Live your life on your terms

- Have interest in other people and stay connected
- Respect your body, it's your temple
- Try new things (what have you got to lose?)
- Stop existing and start living
- Socialise as much as possible with family and friends
- Bring touch, hugs, kisses and love back into your life. It makes you feel better and aids with healing
- Go on a holiday, retreat, getaway
- Involve others in your life. Break down the walls
- Go out for dinner
- Catch up with people for a chat
- Go watch a movie
- Go watch a live band or concert
- Got to the theatre
- Go to a football, soccer, cricket, basketball match, any sport of choice
- Remember people and details about their personal life (be excited to see them and be genuine)
- "Don't be a human doing… be a human being"

Some other points to consider…

DO eat **SLOW**:

S – Seasonal

L – Local

O – Organic

W – Wholefoods

DON'T eat **CRAP**:

C – Carbonated drinks

R – Refined sugars

A – Artificial foods

P – Processed foods

Longevity, health and happiness depends on the least amount of variation in your life… volatility is the enemy. Attach a different meaning to the volatility and challenge and don't take it so personally. Recognise the issue, acknowledge what has happened, feel the emotion, learn the lesson from it and move on. I know it's not always that simple, but do your best to follow these rules as they arise and it will allow you to live a much better life.

Don't dwell on the past, it's come and gone. Hold on to the memories but not the regrets. On the other hand, try not to worry about the future as well. It is OK to plan for it and set goals in advance, but we really should be living in the now and being present in everything that we do.

Stress has an enormous impact on your physical and emotional wellbeing and can shorten your quality and length of life. Stress can have a positive or negative effect on the body, depending on how you learn to deal with it. People's perception of stress is different and individuals cope differently based on how they look at it. There's a positive spin or negative spin to every situation.

Stress can be in the form of a chemical, emotional or physical stressor. I've included some examples for your reference:

- Chemical – deodorants, toothpastes, smoking, soft drinks, alcohol, caffeine, air pollution, pesticides, insecticides

- Emotional – financial, relationship, family, job, unemployment, school, perceptions, lifestyle, death, grief

- Physical – birth process, poor diet, dehydration, lack of exercise (being sedentary), phones and tablets (technology), poor posture (causing pain and discomfort), biochemical, hormones, body's ability to clear toxins, immune system, metabolism, lack of sleep

Something as a simple as a 30-minute walk can reduce stress levels by 50%. It is also important to get some sunlight (Vitamin D) for 15–20 minutes a day, which will allow your body to produce melatonin, helping you to sleep better at night.

Food can trigger certain responses in the body. Everybody reacts differently to different foods, so it's not 'one size fits all' for what you should eat. Listen to your body. It gives you warning signs when something is not quite right. Try taking out certain foods from your diet and reintroduce them again gradually one by one to help you determine which ones may be causing the negative reaction. If you find this too challenging, then please consult a health professional.

In today's society there is a pretence to be happy all of the time. We are human beings with feelings and emotions. It is OK to have mood swings. We need to experience all emotions, from the highs to the lows and find a balance.

We also need to slow down and take time out. Everyone is so busy these days and brags about how busy they are like it's a badge of honour. Introduce more peace and calm into your life by quietening the mind to re-energise and recharge. You should have balance in every area of your life. It will help you feel good on the inside and look good on the outside.

Our character is forged through difficult times and adversity, and through this comes great strength, just as the strongest steel is forged in the hottest fires and diamonds are formed under immense pressure. We all have struggles and challenges at various stages of our life, but you can't become the best version of yourself until you go into the unknown. It shouldn't define you, but rather make you who you are, so don't play the victim.

Lisa and I look at life through very different eyes now and we appreciate things a lot more. It has also changed us as people, for the better. Count your blessings and be grateful and thankful for what you have, not what you don't have. It shouldn't take a life-changing or traumatic event to make you realise what really matters in your life. Work out what your values and beliefs are and what's important to you. These can however change over time and that is fine. It just means that you are growing and evolving as a person.

Have passion and enthusiasm with whatever you do. It's not what you do, but it's how you do it. Do what you love and be your best and you will live a fulfilled life without regrets. Be the best version of you and true to yourself. You are who you are so always remain authentic. Don't be average or mediocre… be the exception to the norm.

Your self-talk and inner thoughts can not only affect your mood, but dictate how people perceive you. Be transparent with your openness and honesty, even if you have to show your vulnerable side. Have a positive mental attitude and be energetic, which in turn will lift people up around you and they will naturally gravitate towards you and your zest for life. Be happy and smile… it's not that hard!

Show empathy towards others and be aware of their feelings by putting yourself in their shoes. Be kind to others and be giving, in both a charitable sense and of yourself. Always remain humble and continue to learn and grow as an individual, partner and family member. Be open to new things and new ideas by surrounding yourself with good people that will challenge you and stretch your way of thinking. But more importantly, look after yourself in every sense of the word. You are GREAT and can have anything that your heart desires.

CHAPTER 16

SO WHAT DOES IT ALL MEAN?

A MUM'S PERSPECTIVE

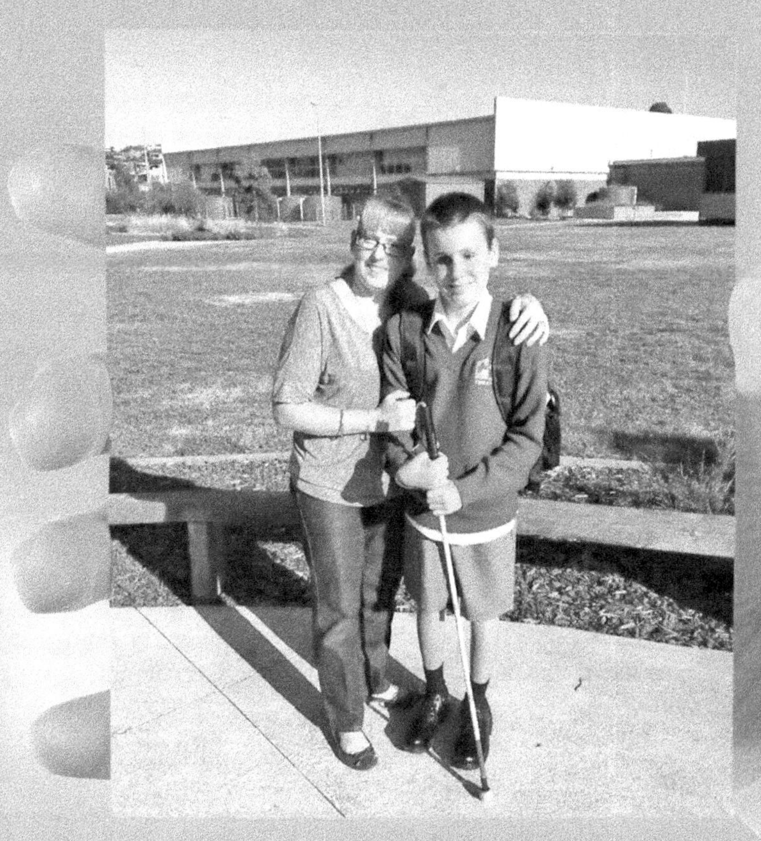

Chapter 16

So What Does It All Mean?

A Mum's Perspective

(Lisa)

> *We must be willing to leave behind the life that we planned so as to have the life that is waiting for us.*
>
> **Joseph Campbell**

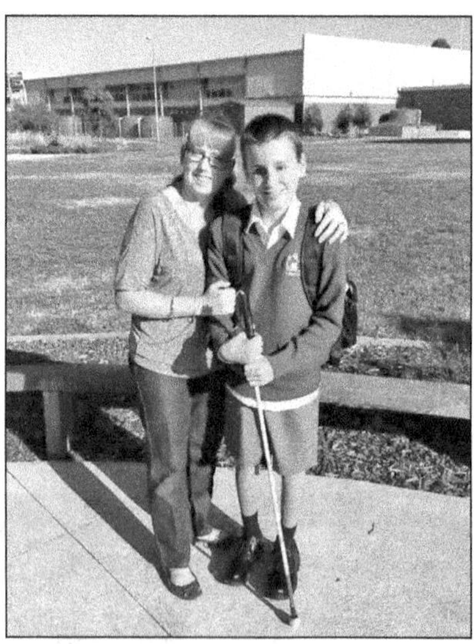

"Everything happens for a reason." Whenever I hear that statement from anybody I just want to slap them! Jim looks at things this way, but I definitely do not. What is the reason for giving a baby cancer before it is even born? What is the reason from letting a father die from cancer, taking him away from a wife and young children? What is the reason for letting kids die before they get a chance to really live?

I do however realise that we all need to make the most of what we are dealt in life. Unfortunately, crap things happen to us all, whether it's big or small. How we all deal with what we are given is up to us. My Mum used to say to me that she didn't know how I coped with all that was happening while Sam was going through treatment. "I have no choice" was my reply. I couldn't give up on Sam, he was my son.

Occasionally I will think back to the details of what we put Sam through, the hospital trips, the pain, the trauma and ultimately the eternal darkness. Depends on where I am emotionally at the time, I still really struggle to this day. And on particularly dark days, I question what kind of Mum I was to give my son cancer while he was inside me.

I know that my emotional struggles sometimes, even to me, seem totally stupid and irrational, but it does not stop them from coming to the surface from time to time.

However, it is a totally different story on my good days.

Don't get me wrong, if I could take away all the life lessons that I have learnt throughout all of this and not have Sam been diagnosed with cancer and been through any of this, I would. Basically, it all sucks. It's not fair what happened to my baby. None of it is fair. I would never wish what has happened to us upon anybody. But it did happen, to Sam and to us. So we had to make the best of a very bad situation. I know that what has happened to Sam and our family has most definitely changed the person who I am. I would not have previously called myself shallow, but I know that my priorities in life and what is important to me has changed. I now look at life through different eyes, pardon the pun.

I sometimes now find it quite funny to watch and observe other people, to see what they think is important. Although I know that everybody's individual issues are important to them, I see things in a whole different way now.

I remember walking around the Royal Children's Hospital, not long after Sam was diagnosed. I remember seeing a young girl who was there, realising that her life would not ever be more than what I was seeing in front of me. Later looking back, she made me feel so incredibly lucky. I realised that Sam had so much life ahead of him. He would be cured of the cancer. He would be blind, but he had a fully functional brain. He still had so much life and so many opportunities ahead of him. He and we were so lucky.

Like people say, there is always someone out there worse off than you. I know that a lot of people say that without really thinking about it, but I realise it every day. I think that people who are the 'Woe is Me' type, need to take a walk around any children's hospital and see what life is really all about and the real problems of the world. It is such a wakeup call.

So, where to from here? That's the million-dollar question. Do any of us really know what lies ahead for us in this game called life? If this wild ride has taught me anything it is to take notice of all those annoying sayings that pop up everywhere. We all know the ones, they say things about making the most of every day, tomorrow is not definite, tell people you love them while you can as you never know if it may be the last time, use the things you keep for 'best' now. These little words of wisdom do seem a bit cheesy, but they are all so true.

And Sam, what does the future hold for this young man, who was behind the eight ball from birth? The thoughts race around my head with this question every day.

I fear the negative. I have heard of many people who were diagnosed with retinoblastoma as young children who survived, only to then suffer a secondary cancer later in life, even into adulthood, and to die from that. I worry that this may be Sam's fate. The fact that he has the retinoblastoma cancer gene, plus all the cancer treatments that he has undergone, especially chemotherapy and radiation, has increased his risk of developing secondary cancers. Ask anybody who knows me, I am a panicky Mum. I always say that I am going to break my neck jumping to conclusions. He has a headache or a sore leg and I hit the panic button. I try to get a balance between paranoia and chilled out, but some days it's damn hard.

Then there are the positives. I see Sam being an inspirational adult. He is an extremely strong willed boy, which, as a 13-year-old is really hard to deal with right now, but shows me that he will get what he wants out of life. I can imagine, as a blind adult, people will tell him he can't do certain things. I can already hear his reply, "Watch me!" Even at his age now, I have witnessed how much he inspires others, even those three or four times his age. I unfortunately quite often now take for granted Sam's amazing abilities, spirit and zest for life. It is when I see him do what he does and people tell me how much they are spurred on by being with Sam, that I sit back, watch him, and regain my admiration for him all over again.

So, where to for Sam? Who knows. All I know is that he will grab whatever life throws at him and run with it. He will continue to do my head in and be a ratty teenager. He will cause me stress and worry. He will make me cry. But he will also make me laugh, bring me joy and happiness. He will continue to make me proud of him, I will continue to be in awe of my son. But most of all, I will always be grateful that he entered my life, and that he is who he is. I am privileged to be Sam's Mum.

Samuel Valavanis. Watch this space…

CHAPTER 17

SAM... MY INSPIRATION

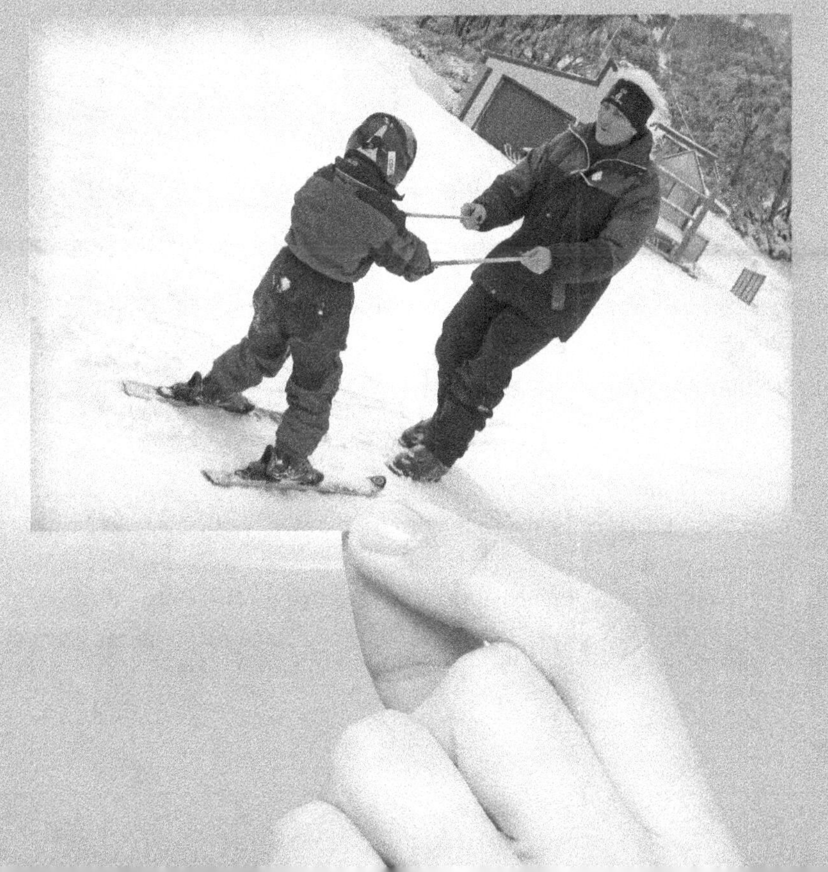

Chapter 17

Sam... My Inspiration

(Jim)

> *We cannot choose our external circumstances, but we can always choose how we respond to them.*
>
> **Epictetus**

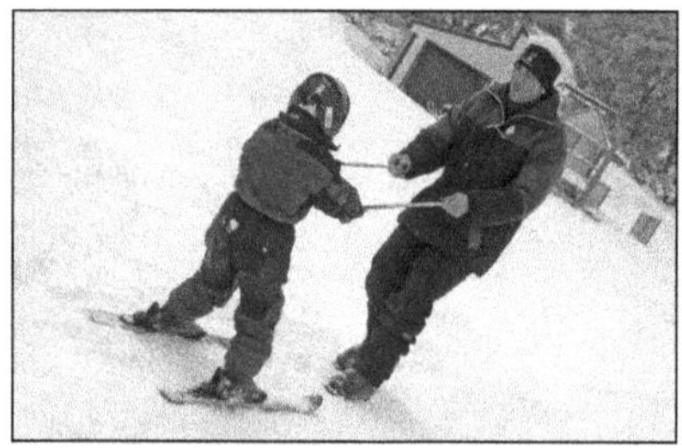

As difficult as it has been to share our family's personal journey throughout this book, there are a number of reasons that we have chosen to go down this path. We have been fortunate enough to come out of this whole ordeal with a bright, funny and inquisitive boy we still have in our lives, who has taught us the true meaning of life.

Some time ago I was sitting in a food court having my lunch watching a mother with her little girl that had Down's Syndrome and was totally overcome with emotions, to the point where I had tears in my eyes. She was being so gentle and patient with her that it touched me. I believe that it is true when they say someone upstairs gives special kids to special people and we are never given more than we can handle. I didn't understand this at first but it has hit home more recently and rings true.

Our main reasons for sharing our story are...

- To raise awareness of retinoblastoma and educate parents on the warning signs to look for
- To let parents and loved ones know that there is light at the end of the tunnel
- To show that you can bounce back and break through from the depths of despair to live a joyous and fulfilling life
- To know how to overcome adversity when faced with a life changing event
- To help children cope with grief and loss and move on
- To understand how the power of positive thinking can help you heal following a traumatic event
- To recognise the signs of anxiety and depression and work through it with the right advice and help (and to know where to find it)
- To raise much needed funds and awareness for charities like the Starlight Children's Foundation and other amazing organisations
- To learn how to come to terms with your child having a disability and what that means for their future
- To offer a sense of hope and inspiration to people going through tough times in their lives

We don't give Sam any special treatment or leniency compared to his brother and sister. He is 'normal' to us in every way. We definitely don't wrap Sam up in cottonwool and hide him away in a corner. We encourage him to be independent and try new things all the time. He is very adventurous and has no fear, which will take him to places far and wide, enabling him to meet some extraordinary people around the world.

We don't see him as a disabled child, nor do we like to use that term. Disabled means unable to do things… the only thing he can't do is see. But when you watch him getting around and climbing all over the playgrounds, you begin to question whether he is actually blind. We will quite often get asked, "How much can he see?" It's a bit of a shock to other people when we answer with, "Nothing, he's had both eyes removed!"

Most of our lessons in life have come through struggles, difficult times, adversity and challenges. It helps you put things into perspective and work out what's really important, and be grateful for everything that you have in your life. We as a family have never had the victim mentality or asked, "Why us?" There are two paths you can consciously choose to take; you can play the victim and let it dictate and rule your life and keep you in a negative state of mind, or you can be the victor and take ownership of the situation and learn to accept what has happened, and hopefully one day your story will inspire others to live life to the best of their ability.,

Sam has had a pretty good run since his remission in 2007, which we have been truly thankful for. However, 2014 was a year that saw us make countless trips to the GP. Sam even had an admission to hospital with a recurring kidney and urinary tract infection. But with all this time in the waiting room more recently it brought back the memories of what we went through for four and a half years. In the back of your mind we were thinking to ourselves; has it returned, could it be a secondary tumour, is it related to the treatments we subjected him to? It plays with your head and I don't know if I'll ever be able to get over it.

I still don't know how we did it, especially Lisa who was there for most of the hospital trips and treatment. It was like we were on autopilot and only focussing on what needed to be done to get Sam better. Looking back on it now, it was all a blur and we were living week to week and month to month.

We had amazing support from family and friends, who would do whatever they could to help us through these very difficult times, including bringing us meals, running errands, picking up kids or babysitting for us. We were also fortunate enough to meet some wonderful staff and other parents at the hospital with whom we still stay in contact with today.

We are extremely lucky to be living in Melbourne and have the Royal Children's Hospital on our doorstep, which is world class with its medical staff, research and treatment. The Doctors and staff were exceptional from the moment we first arrived in November 2002, and we couldn't speak more highly of them. They couldn't do enough for us and made Sam feel very special. It was like a second home to us during that period, between 2002 to 2007, and Sam describes it to this day as his 'Luna Park'! He still looks forward to his return visits and has to do a tour each time we go in and say hi to as many people as he can. It has had a significant impact on him.

As much as I would like to have a 'normal family and do normal family things, we just have to realise that this will not always be possible. Something as simple as jumping in the car and going on a family outing for the day has to be pre-planned and thought through, to ensure that Sam will be able to participate and get the most out of the experience. We don't take things for granted but appreciate that he is keen and willing to make it a memorable experience for all of us.

The future for Sam...

In our darkest hours it was very hard to see the light at the end of the tunnel, but today I see a very bright future for Sam. He has been through a lot in his short life and with everything he has endured it has made him a very strong willed, resilient and determined boy who can tackle anything that is thrown at him. He is a perfectionist in everything he does, which can frustrate him (and us) at times, but the main thing is he will give it a go.

Sam has a wonderful imagination and can paint a very colourful and vivid picture in his mind of the world around him. He is extremely creative and a great story teller which comes from listening to a broad range of audio books and DVD's. He plays out scenes with his toys and brings them to life, entertaining himself for hours on end.

His music teacher indicated to us that he has perfect pitch and has been given a gift. She would play a musical piece or he would hear a song on the radio and be able to play it back to you without much thought. It just came naturally to him, so I hope that he continues his love of music as he gets older. After all, music is an international language. When he first started playing, he told us that he wanted to learn as many musical instruments as possible. He has since changed his mind now that he knows how much work and practice it takes.

He has an amazing memory for dates and numbers. If you were to introduce him to a new person, the next time he saw them he would be able to tell you their full name, address, phone number etc. He memorises songs, artists and which disc they were on and in what particular order. If only he was that good with the lotto numbers! He also remembers things he did on certain dates. Another freaky thing we have worked out is that he can tell you the days of the week a particular date falls on. He is our 'Rain Man'!

Sam is a very intelligent boy and has a hunger for knowledge and learning. His curiosity has him questioning things all the time until he finds the answers or facts, which he will amazingly retain for future reference when needed. He is already telling us that he wants to become an Anaesthetist when he grows up, to help others like they have helped him since he was only twelve weeks old.

Sam can certainly teach us all a thing or two about the little things we take for granted. Whether it be tying your shoelaces or brushing your teeth, he doesn't let it get him down and sees it as a challenge more than anything. He is a great example of an individual that has overcome adversity with what life has thrown at him and made the most of his situation.

The fact that Sam is vision impaired does not restrict him to a sedate and slow paced lifestyle. In actual fact, it's quite the opposite. He loves adventure, thrill rides, outdoor activities and anything that will test him physically. This drive and sense of wanting more out of life gives us comfort in knowing that Sam will strive to be the best he can be, sighted or not. The character traits he possesses at this early age draw people to him and this pushes him to want to do more and achieve more.

We are quite often asked if Sam will have a Guide Dog when he gets older. It was hard enough to get him to use a cane when he lost his sight, which we have named "Michael" (aka Michael Caine, the actor) to give it a personality rather than just being an object! He feels that the cane draws attention to him and labels him as blind and disabled. He longs more than ever to be like all of the other children. At this stage I'm not convinced that he will have a Guide Dog, but never say never. He says that they are dirty, smelly and slobber all over you, but I feel that a dog would make a great companion for him and give him far more independence than he realises.

Sam has an Orientation and Mobility Instructor who teaches him to get out and about on his own. He was taught to walk to school and navigate his way around the campus without the need for an Aid or assistance from others. Another skill which he has mastered from a young age is the ability to map out new places in his mind. He will work out where the perimeters are and then determine the location of objects within those perimeters. Once he has done this he feels confident in getting around unassisted. It is very interesting to watch. This will hold him in good stead in his adult life as he navigates his way around town and utilises public transport, which he already loves doing.

He also uses another self-taught skill called 'echolocation', where he will click his tongue on the roof of his mouth. (Wikipedia: Human echolocation is an ability of humans to detect objects in their environment by sensing echoes from those objects. By actively creating sounds – for example, by tapping their canes, lightly stomping their feet, snapping their fingers, or making clicking noises with their mouths – people trained to orient by echolocation can interpret the sound waves reflected by nearby objects, accurately identifying their location and size).

He attends support skills twice a term at the Statewide Vision Resource Centre (SVRC), where they assist him with life skills and independence, which he is extremely determined to achieve sooner rather than later.

If ever there was a time to be living with a vision impairment, then this certainly is the right era, with all of the advancements in modern medicine and technology. From a Braille Note to a personal GPS watch, from early diagnosis and less invasive treatments to bionic eyes. We are seeing things move so fast these days and I would like to live in the hope and belief that he will see our faces again in his lifetime, whether they be pixelated or not.

Sam has taught us so much about what's really important in life and to look at the world through different eyes. These valuable life lessons have allowed us to reprioritise what is important to us as individuals and as a family, our goals and plans for the future, and to look ahead now more than ever, ready to experience everything that comes our way with a positive attitude.

Whether you got cut off by somebody in traffic on the way to work, or your cup of coffee you bought wasn't hot enough, it isn't life changing, so you need to put everything into perspective and ask yourself, "Is this really going to drastically change my life?"

He has shown us that we all need to live life to the fullest and cherish each day. Go on that family holiday that you keep postponing, try something new that you would never have done in a million years, tell the people close to you how much they mean to you and do something special for them.

We live in such a fast-paced world today where time will pass you by in the blink of an eye. We need to take a step back and "smell the roses" and live in the now. Social and economic pressures are forcing us to keep up with the Joneses and have all the unnecessary luxuries. These are all materialistic things and at the end of the day they don't really make us any happier in the long term. They are a quick fix to give us instant gratification.

Why not give some money to a charity, donate some toys or clothes to the needy, or even better still, give up your time to assist those that are doing it tough? It is so much more rewarding to see a smile on someone's face or to get a hug off somebody that you've never met before, but who's life you have been able to change for the better in some way, whether it be big or small.

I truly believe that what has happened to us with Sam has happened for a reason, and he is here as an example to others of what one can do with positive reinforcement and a "can do" attitude.

No matter what your physical or mental disability or handicap, you should not be pigeonholed and wrapped in cottonwool to live your life on welfare support. We have encouraged Sam to follow his dreams and to be the best person he can be and not let obstacles get in his way, both physically and metaphorically.

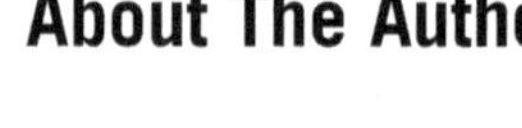

About The Authors

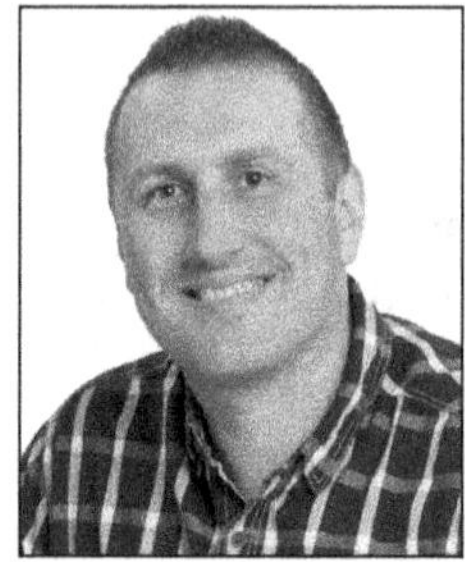

Jim Valavanis

International Author, Speaker and Parent

Jim is an author, parent and inspirational public speaker on overcoming daunting adversities in family life and how we can benefit and empower ourselves and others by changing negative expectations of just *'surviving'* life's challenges to *'thriving'* in life's challenges.

He is the International author of ***Life Through Sam's Eyes – How our Blind Son Helped Us See.***

Jim has shared with many the moving and inspiring story of how his son, Sam, was diagnosed with retinoblastoma (eye cancer) and how he and his wife, Lisa, not only coped with confronting and difficult circumstances, but how they became more resilient, created a positive environment and a compelling future not just for Sam, but for the family as a whole.

He's been involved with many charitable organisations such as Beyond Sight Auxiliary, Royal Children's Hospital Good Friday Appeal, Starlight Children's Foundation, Camp Quality, Challenge, Ronald McDonald House Charities, Cancer Council, Guide Dogs and Vision Australia.

Jim has a diverse range of qualifications that has bridged over two decades including Sports Medicine, Massage, Football Trainer, Real Estate, Sales Consultant, Business Development Manager and his most important role yet… Parent!

Jim's association and participation with a variety of sporting institutions and organisations over the years including cricket, football, basketball, soccer, running, cycling, golf, taekwondo and kung fu has contributed greatly to his appreciation and need for persistence and tenacity in all facets of life.

He has travelled extensively to numerous countries around the world, including the United States of America, Greece, Turkey, Mexico, Fiji and Philippines, just to name a few.

Jim lives in Melbourne, Australia with his wife Lisa and their 3 children, Samuel, Mitchell and Caitlin.

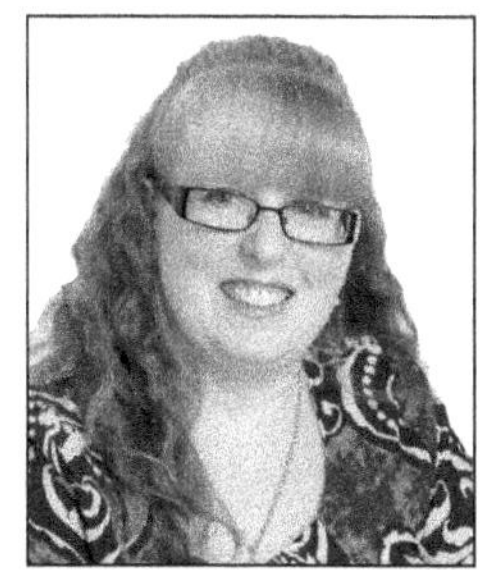

Lisa Valavanis

International Author, Speaker and Parent.

Lisa is an author, parent and inspiring speaker on tackling life's difficulties head-on. Providing inspiration to all on how seeming insurmountable obstacles can be met and ultimately mastered.

She is the International author of **Life Through Sam's Eyes** – ***How our Blind Son Helped Us See.***

Lisa has shared her family's heart wrenching ordeal openly, telling of her young son's experience with challenging odds, helping many families and individuals through traumatic experiences and giving direction and hope for the future.

Lisa's appearances on many television programs, radio, newspapers and magazines nationally have told of her family's journey from devastation to inspiration.

She has travelled the world extensively, including places such as England, the United States of America, Mexico, Fiji and New Zealand, just to name a few.

As a philanthropist, Lisa has been involved with various charitable organisations such as Beyond Sight Auxiliary, Vision Australia, Rotary, Starlight Children's Foundation, Camp Quality, Challenge, Ronald McDonald House Charities, Guide Dogs, Royal Children's Hospital Good Friday Appeal, Cancer Council and various other fundraising committees.

Through her self-taught Event Management skills, Lisa has organised and held two Beyond Sight Family Fun Days, raising in excess of $30,000 for the Beyond Sight Auxiliary.

Lisa has also previously held the leadership role of School Council President at her sons' Primary School for three consecutive years.

After 16 years of working in the Health Industry, Lisa has decided it is now time to steer her life in a new direction and focus on what is important to her.

Lisa lives in Melbourne, Australia with her husband Jim and their 3 children Samuel, Mitchell and Caitlin.

Social Media and Contact Details

Jim

Jim Valavanis (Author)

Jim Valavanis

jimvalavanis

Jim Valavanis

Jim Valavanis

@jimvalavanis

Jim Valavanis

Lisa

Lisa Valavanis (Author)

Lisa Valavanis

lisavalavanis

Lisa Valavanis

Lisa Valavanis

@lisaValavanis

Lisa Valavanis

Other

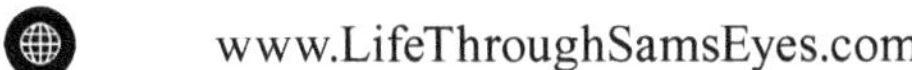

www.LifeThroughSamsEyes.com

lifethroughsamseyes@gmail.com

Life Through Sam's Eyes

Dragonfly Connection

Live Life At 100

Life Through Sam's Eyes (Blog)

Life Through Sam's Eyes

Live Life At 100 (Podcast)

RESOURCE DIRECTORY

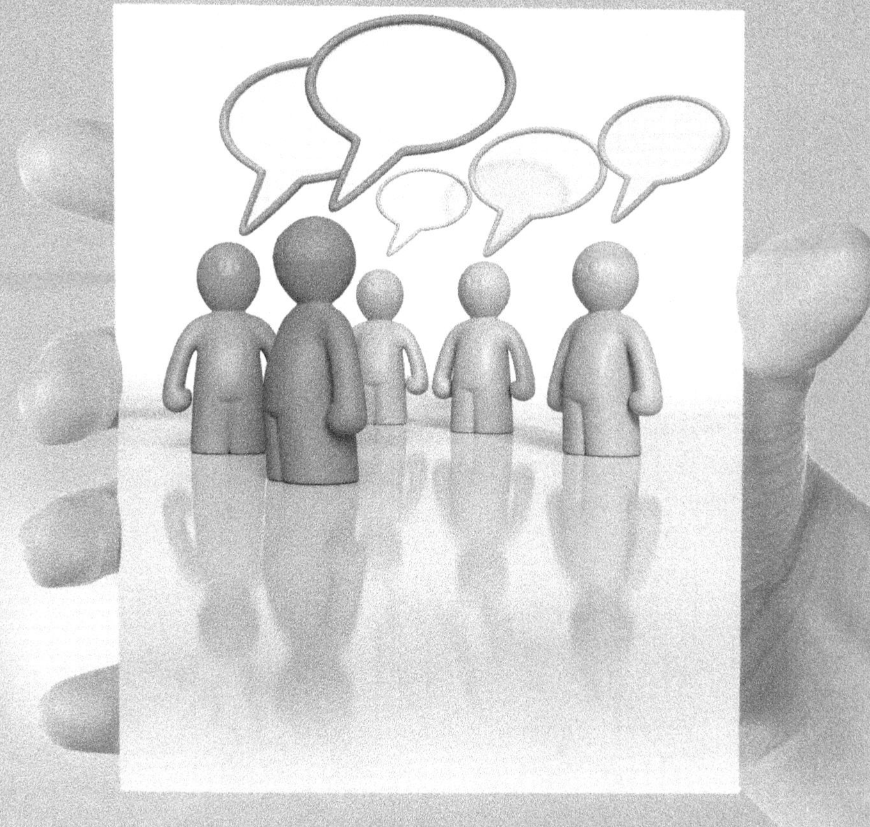

Resource Directory

Charities

- **Beyond Sight – Royal Children's Hospital Auxiliary**
  The Royal Children's Hospital Foundation
  Level 2, 48 Flemington Road
  Parkville VIC 3052
  Phone: (03) 9345 5037
  Website: www.foundation.rch.org.au/?page=Auxiliaries-Beyond-Sight

- **Camp Quality Limited**
  Suite 6, 44-46 Oxford Street
  Epping NSW 2121
  Phone: (02) 9876 0500
  Website: www.campquality.org.au

- **CanTeen**
  161 Flemington Road
  North Melbourne VIC 3051
  Phone: 1800 226 833
  Website: www.canteen.org.au

- **Challenge**
  529-535 King Street
  West Melbourne VIC 3003
  Phone: (03) 9329 8474
  Website: www.challenge.org.au

- **Clown Doctors – The Humour Foundation**
  Level 1, 28 Bridge Street
  Pymble NSW 2073
  Phone: 1300 486 687
  Website: www.humourfoundation.com.au

- **Make-A-Wish Australia**
  1/620 Church Street
  Richmond VIC 3121
  Phone: 1800 032 260
  Website: www.makeawish.org.au

- **Redkite (formerly Malcolm Sargent Cancer Fund For Children)**
  Level 8, Tower 1, 1 Lawson Square
  Redfern NSW 2016
  Phone: (02) 9219 4000
  Website: www.redkite.org.au

- **Ronald McDonald House Charities**
  21-29 Central Ave
  Thornleigh NSW 2120
  Phone: (02) 9875 6666
  Website: www.rmhc.org.au

- **Starlight Children's Foundation**
  Level 3, 80 Chandos Street
  Naremburn NSW 2065
  Phone: 1300 727 827
  Website: www.starlight.org.au

- **Variety Australia – The Children's Charity**
  47 Herbert Street
  Artarmon NSW 2064
  Phone: (02) 9819 1001
  Website: www.variety.org.au

- **Very Special Kids**
  321 Glenferrie Road
  Malvern VIC 3144
  Phone: 1800 888 875
  Website: www.vsk.org.au

Cancer Support/Services

- **Australian Cancer Research Foundation**
  Suite 409, The Strand Arcade
  412 George Street
  Sydney NSW 2000
  Phone: (02) 9223 7833
  Website: www.acrf.com.au

- **Cancer Council Australia**
  Level 14, 477 Pitt Street
  Sydney NSW 2000
  Phone: 13 11 20
  Website: www.cancer.org.au

- **Kids with Cancer Foundation Australia**
  22/22 Hudson Avenue
  Castle Hill NSW 2154
  Phone: 1800 255 522
  Website: www.kidswithcancer.org.au

- **Murdoch Children's Research Institute**
  Royal Children's Hospital
  Flemington Road
  Parkville VIC 3052
  Phone: 1300 766 439
  Website: www.mcri.edu.au

- **Peter MacCallum Cancer Foundation**
  Level 6 , 372 Albert Street
  East Melbourne VIC 3002
  Phone: 1800 111 440
  Website: www.foundation.petermac.org

Vision Services

- **Blind Sports Victoria**
  454 Glenferrie Road
  Kooyong VIC 3144
  Phone: (03) 9822 8876
  Website: www.blindsports.org.au

- **Bolinda Publishing – Audio Books**
  17 Mohr Street
  Tullamarine VIC 3043
  Phone: (03) 9338 0666
  Website: www.bolinda.com/aus

- **Guide Dogs Australia**
  Phone: 1800 484 333
  Website: www.guidedogsaustralia.com

- **Guide Dogs Victoria**
  2-6 Chandler Highway
  Kew VIC 3101
  Phone: 1800 804 805
  Website: www.guidedogsvictoria.com.au

- **Insight Education Centre for the Blind and Vision Impaired**
  120 Enterprise Avenue
  Berwick VIC 3806
  Phone: 1800 474 448
  Website: www.insightvision.org.au

- **Royal Institute for Deaf and Blind Children (RIDBC)**
  361-365 North Rocks Road
  North Rocks NSW 2151
  Phone: (02) 9871 1233
  Website: www.ridbc.org.au

- **Seeing Eye Dogs Australia**
  17 Barrett Street
  Kensington VIC 3031
  Phone: 1800 037 773
  Website: www.seda.visionaustralia.org

- **Statewide Vision Resource Centre**
  370 Springvale Road
  Donvale VIC 3111
  Phone: (03) 9841 0242
  Website: www.svrc.vic.edu.au

- **Vision Australia (formerly RVIB)**
  454 Glenferrie Road
  Kooyong VIC 3144
  Phone: 1300 847 466
  Website: www.visionaustralia.org

- **Feelix Library – Vision Australia**
  454 Glenferrie Road
  Kooyong VIC 3144
  Phone: 1300 847 466
  Website: www.visionaustralia.org/living-with-low-vision/library/feelix-library

- **Vision 2020 Australia**
  Level 2, 174 Queen Street
  Melbourne VIC 3000
  Phone: (03) 9656 2020
  Website: www.vision2020australia.org.au

Disability Services / Respite Services

- **Bestchance - Child Family Care**
  583 Ferntree Gully Road
  Glen Waverley VIC 3150
  Phone: (03) 8202 8308
  Website: www.bestchance.org.au

- **Department of Health & Human Services**
  50 Lonsdale Street
  Melbourne VIC 3000
  Phone: 1300 650 172
  Website: www.humanservices.gov.au or
  www.dhs.vic.gov.au/for-individuals/disability/carer-and-family-support/respite-support-information

- **MOIRA Disability & Youth Services**
  928 Nepean Highway
  Hampton East VIC 3188
  Phone: 03) 8552 2222
  Website: www.moira.org.au

- **Respite Victoria**
  Phone: 1800 052 222
  Website: www.respitevictoria.org.au or
  www.carersvictoria.org.au/advice/services-supports/respite-carer-support

- **Scope (Vic)**
  830 Whitehorse Road
  Box Hill VIC 3128
  Phone: 1300 472 673
  Website: www.scopevic.org.au

- **Villa Maria Catholic Homes**
  486 Albert Street
  East Melbourne VIC 3002
  Phone: 1800 036 377
  Website: www.vmch.com.au

- **Yooralla**
  Level 14, 595 Collins Street
  Melbourne Victoria 3000
  Phone: (03) 9666 4500
  Website: www.yooralla.com.au

Mental Health Support / Services

- **Beyond Blue**
  Level 1, 40 Burwood Road
  Hawthorn VIC 3122
  Phone: 1300 224 636
  Website: www.beyondblue.org.au

- **Black Dog Institute**
  Hospital Road
  Prince of Wales Hospital
  Randwick NSW 2031
  Reception/General Information: (02) 9382 4530
  Clinics: (02) 9382 2991
  Website: www.blackdoginstitute.org.au

- **Headspace**
  Level 2, South Tower
  485 La Trobe Street
  Melbourne VIC 3000
  Phone: (03) 9027 0100
  Website: www.headspace.org.au

- **Kids Helpline**
  GPO Box 2469
  Brisbane QLD 4001
  Phone: 1800 551 800
  Website: www.kidshelpline.com.au

- **Lifeline**
  PO Box 173
  Deakin ACT 2600
  Phone: 13 11 14
  Website: www.lifeline.org.au

- **MensLine Australia**
  PO Box 2335
  Footscray VIC 3011
  Phone: 1300 789 978
  Website: www.mensline.org.au

- **The Reach Foundation**
  152-156 Wellington Street
  Collingwood VIC 3066
  Phone: (03) 9412 0900
  Website: www.reach.org.au

www.ingramcontent.com/pod-product-compliance
Lightning Source LLC
Chambersburg PA
CBHW060615290326
41930CB00051B/1830
* 9 7 8 1 9 2 2 1 1 8 6 7 7 *